P9-CBC-124

the PRACTITIONER'S CREDO

To Eric,

Good luck in your efforts for the professions. Hope you enjoy the read.

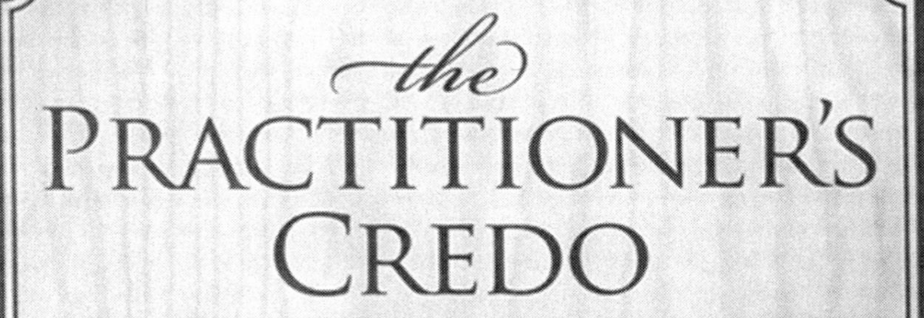

DR. JOHN B. MATTINGLY, DMD, MS

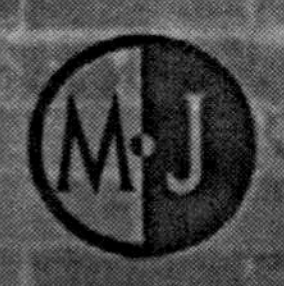

New York

The Practitioner's Credo

10 Keys to a Successful Practice

Copyright 2009 John Mattingly. All rights reserved.

No part of this publication may be reproduced or transmitted in any form or by any means, mechanical or electronic, including photocopying and recording, or by any information storage and retrieval system, without permission in writing from the author or publisher (except by a reviewer, who may quote brief passages and/or short brief video clips in a review.)

Disclaimer: The Publisher and the Author make no representations or warranties with respect to the accuracy or completeness of the contents of this work and specifically disclaim all warranties, including without limitation warranties of fitness for a particular purpose. No warranty may be created or extended by sales or promotional materials. The advice and strategies contained herein may not be suitable for every situation. This work is sold with the understanding that the Publisher is not engaged in rendering legal, accounting, or other professional services. If professional assistance is required, the services of a competent professional person should be sought. Neither the Publisher nor the Author shall be liable for damages arising herefrom. The fact that an organization or website is referred to in this work as a citation and/or a potential source of further information does not mean that the Author or the Publisher endorses the information the organization or website may provide or recommendations it may make. Further, readers should be aware that internet websites listed in this work may have changed or disappeared between when this work was written and when it is read.

Paperback ISBN: 978-1-60037-556-9

Hardcover ISBN: 978-1-60037-557-6

Library of Congress Control Number: 2008943940

MORGAN · JAMES
THE ENTREPRENEURIAL PUBLISHER

Morgan James Publishing, LLC
1225 Franklin Ave., STE 325
Garden City, NY 11530-1693
Toll Free 800-485-4943
www.MorganJamesPublishing.com

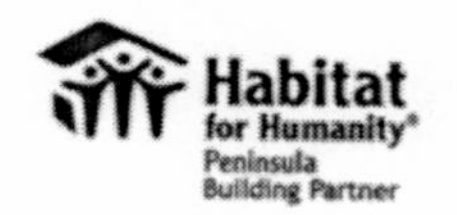

In an effort to support local communities, raise awareness and funds, Morgan James Publishing donates one percent of all book sales for the life of each book to Habitat for Humanity. Get involved today, visit **www.HelpHabitatForHumanity.org.**

Table of Contents

Prologue

Probably before elaborating on what I consider the ten Keys to a successful practice, a brief discussion of the evolution of "our" practice and how we relate to team members is in order at this time. When I first started in practice 34 years ago and the practice gradually grew from one staff member to the current 26 team members, it was similar to opening a book in the middle.

I was born the second of six children, my father a construction electrician and my mother a school teacher by training. My older brother died of spinal meningitis as an infant. When I was five years of age, our parents moved me and my three brothers and one sister from Hawesville, Kentucky to Louisville in search of better job opportunities. My sister joined the convent one year out of high school and is still a Maryknoll Nun. My three younger brothers, all of whom served in the U. S. Army during the Vietnam War, are union electricians. I did not complete post-graduate training and start practicing orthodontics until I was 31 years of age. I had received a Bachelor's Degree with a major in chemistry (University of Louisville, 1961), worked two years at Sinclair Research Labs in Harvey, Illinois (during which time I married Joyce Daniels – a Louisville sweetheart), then returned to Louisville where I attended and graduated from dental school (University of Louisville Dental School, 1967). I subsequently enlisted in the military (served as Capt. U.S. Air Force Dental Corps, stationed on Guam from 1967-69), primarily because of respectful regard for my repeated reclassifications as 2S (student deferment) which allowed me to complete my schooling while all my brothers and many of my friends were drafted into the military during the Vietnam War. After the Vietnam War wound down and I completed my tour of duty, I entered specialty orthodontic training and graduated from Northwestern University Dental School in Chicago, 1971. I had never taken a business course in all this schooling, except for two classes at the University of Chicago MBA

Program night school, in 1962, where I was overwhelmed, and decided I had better stick to a science curriculum. To this day, I have regretted my lack of business training.

Joyce and I and our two young children moved back to Louisville following graduation from the orthodontic residency program at Northwestern, rented an apartment and opened an orthodontic practice. I worked two days a week for another practitioner on the other side of town and saw patients the other three weekdays and Saturday mornings at my practice location.

I initially hired only a receptionist who answered the occasional phone call at our 1,000 square foot office, and where she spent a great deal of time reading the Bible while waiting for the phone to ring. As the practice began to build, I next employed an 18-year old recent high school graduate who later confided about "fudging" her age. But, she was just what the practice needed ... energetic, bright, effervescent, friendly, and extremely outgoing. After being with us for seven years, she eventually married an Air Force officer and has remained a friend to this day. That was over 30 years ago, and she is still working in an orthodontic office. She has been employed as an orthodontic assistant in California, Germany, Italy, Virginia, Florida -- wherever her husband was stationed. Her husband gradually climbed the promotion ladder to full "Bird" Colonel so the role of money was not her primary motivating factor. She takes pride in her abilities and excels at the role of team player. We have been their houseguests in Germany, Italy, California, and Florida and still remain in close touch.

As the practice gradually developed and we took on more staff members, our initial efforts at building a camaraderie of spirit among team members was to go out for an occasional lunch together. Or, sometimes, we would gather for a beer or glass of wine on Friday afternoon after work at a neighborhood pub across the street from our practice. The practice has now evolved to the point where we have regular family activities such as renting out a 12 lane bowling alley from 6:00-10:00pm for team members' families with soft drinks, beer and fried bologna sandwiches provided ... or a night at the ball park for team members, spouses and kids, day at the horse races, etc. All of these family activities, we feel, are an integral part of our practice. They allow us to know and appreciate our team members, their spouses and their families. Team leaders and team members alike attend weddings, kids' athletic events and the celebration of new life when a team member is blessed with a new baby! We have mandatory staff meetings where all issues are on the table and each section (Lab, Front Desk and Clinic Floor) must make contributions to the agenda. There are currently three team leaders, my son Chris, who has been on board for almost 15 years, and Chris Howell, who joined us approximately seven years ago. Each of us has various strengths, and all are truly team oriented. We meet frequently to discuss procedures, fee schedules, staff meeting topics, discounts, perks, treatment concerns, problems and any other issue that needs to be addressed. There are no topics which are taboo to discuss. Each of us is totally committed to the practice and still we are all family oriented, socially active extroverts. We have all benefited from our practice ties as well as from the special relationship we have with the other team members and their families. We understand and appreciate the necessity to treat team members as family because team members seek this feeling of security and trust as much as anything we can offer them. And when we find a good team member, we strive to keep her/him with us. As of this writing, we currently have 26 staff members including the three team leaders working at our two locations, some of whom are part time while others have chosen to work full time. The choice is theirs to make. Some are high school students working co-op status and are paid on an hourly basis. All personnel working 30 hours or more are considered full time in our practice and are entitled to full time benefits.

Currently, each location of the practice has seven chairs on the clinic floors and an additional 2-3 chairs for records and new patient exams. The satellite office in Bardstown, Kentucky (approximately 40 miles from the Louisville office) was opened in 1992 when my son Chris entered the practice, and he was the primary influence in its development and growth. Since my retirement, Chris Mattingly and

Chris Howell alternate working time in each office, with each office staffed by team members from their respective communities.

The idea for the book you are now reading originated in early 2005, and I began writing at that time. I retired from the practice at the end of that year, and the writing was subsequently completed a few years later. In a progressive practice such as ours, many changes can occur in policy and protocol regularly. Therefore, the office policy manual that was in effect when I retired is updated annually and obviously has changed. However, one thing is constant ... our ongoing efforts to acknowledge our team members as "family" and to treat them accordingly.

The FIRST Key
Practice Leadership

It was former President Harry Truman who said that "The Buck Stops Here." Never was that adage more true than when describing the person or persons whose practice bears their name. The Team Leader/ Leaders are undoubtedly the primary foundation from which any successful practice emanates. They ultimately have the responsibility for everything that goes on in the office as well as what comes out of the office. The type of practice, the type of staff that makes up a practice and even the type of patients who are drawn to the practice are a direct influence of the leadership of the team captains.

If there is one principle that sets the tone for team leaders, a good case could be made for the Golden Rule. "Treat others as you would have them treat you!" Nothing influences staff, patients, colleagues, delivery people, janitors, ad infinitum, more than treating people with respect. There should never be a time when respect is taken for granted and common courtesy not extended. When team members come to work, the complete person comes to work ... that is to say their concerns about their spouses, children, mortgage payments, etc. Some may be concerned about their own or family members' health, school grades or any other countless concerns. It can be readily understood that any team member will have bad days, good days and better days. However, each of us lives by a set of guidelines and, in fact, truly expects and appreciates guidelines. When team members live within practice guidelines, the difference between good days and bad days are blurred. Respect for each other and the duties at hand dictate focus and attention to common etiquette. Therefore, it is an essential characteristic of a team leader that all guidelines issued be fair, consistent and enforced. This also means unequivocal adherence to any established guidelines by the team leader/leaders.

It is my judgment that team leaders must lead by being role models. It is their responsibility to convey to team members, and to everyone with whom they come in contact, that integrity, concern for other people and an uncompromising sense of ethics are personal values that take highest priority. These values should be sincere and consistent. If team members of varied ideologies recognize in the team leaders a consistent sense of ethics, the effects can raise the bar in the office setting and allow all members to realize their maximum potential.

There are some practitioners who charge higher fees if a patient has insurance coverage. There are some practitioners who consider payment of taxes obtrusive and do everything possible to evade paying them. Woe to the practitioner who mistakenly believes that staff is unaware of unscrupulous behavior by the team leader.

The team leader should grant to every member of the team making up the practice the authority to do whatever is in the best interests of the practice and the patients we serve, so long as these actions are legal, ethical and done with the right intentions. A team leader has the obligation to oversee but not to supervise. Micro management is a guaranteed way to undermine creativity and effort. Empowered team members feel a sense of confidence in making decisions beneficial to the practice. There are many times when a group think is not always possible when team members are confronted with something out of the ordinary.

Bearing in mind that the responsibility for everything that goes on in the office as well as what comes out of the office, is borne by the team leader/leaders, everything must be checked, approved and endorsed prior to patient dismissal.

Goals should be established as a team, and all members of the team should have some say in the manner in which the practice is run. A practice is successful when the team feels it is their practice. Patients perceive a practice as being successful not by the amount of advertising the practice does, nor by the splendor of the facility it is housed in, but rather by how the team and team leaders relate to each other and to the patients in their care.

Leadership is the engine that drives one group to excel over another … the motivator that makes one practice more productive than another … and the impetus that takes integrity, ethics and concern for other people to the level that generates success. How many times have you professed loyalty to a brand name, a hotel franchise, a department store or any number of businesses that provide a service that is superior to others in their field? This loyalty was not flippantly placed, but was earned by the businesses' consistent emphasis on extraordinary service and customer satisfaction. In every instance, the effectiveness of the particular business concern in projecting its image of service and customer satisfaction could be traced to the leadership of the organization who has made the conscious decision to emphasize those features and to develop a product along those lines.

This same phenomenon relates as well to any professional practice. It is the team leader's responsibility to convey to team members, colleagues, patients and to any person who has any dealings with the practice, that a consistent sense of excellent service, ethics, and concern for people is intrinsic to the practice and will not be compromised.

This mantle of leadership, which has been earned by virtue of your licensure into a profession, offers the opportunity to conduct your practice in any manner you choose. Your choices will ultimately determine to which level of success your practice gravitates. If your goal is to have a practice which is perceived as successful, is admired by your colleagues, appreciated by your patients and respected by everyone, your choices should be directed toward two-way respect and an equitable and just philosophy of practice administration. Just as loyalty to a given brand name is earned, loyalty to your practice must be earned … but once it is earned, you reap the benefits of people telling other people about their positive experiences. There can be no better marketing mechanism!!!

The FIRST Key – Practice Leadership

- The Team Leader/Leaders are the primary foundation from which any practice emanates.
- The type of practice, the type of staff that makes up a practice, and even the type of patients that are drawn to the practice are a direct result of the leadership of the team captains.
- If there is one adage that sets the tone for team leaders, a good case could be made for "treat others as you would have them treat you!"
- It is an essential characteristic of a team leader that all guidelines issued be fair, consistent and enforced.
- It is the team leader's responsibility to convey to team members, and to everyone they come in contact with, that integrity, concern for other people and an uncompromising sense of ethics are personal values that take the highest priority.
- A practice is successful when the team members feel it is their practice.
- Patients perceive a practice as being successful not by the amount of advertising the practice does, nor by the splendor of the facility it is housed in, but rather by how the team and team leaders relate to each other and to the patients in their care.
- Loyalty to your practice must be earned … but once earned, the practice reaps the benefit of people telling other people of their positive experiences. There can be no better marketing mechanism!

The SECOND Key
Enthusiastic, Effective Staff

It is not without reason that successful practices all enjoy the stability of happy, secure, hard-working staff. This critical stability is what turns a staff into a team and plays an integral part in the success of any practice. Each staff member has individual responsibilities, but all members have to operate with consideration for the best interests of the team and the public we all serve. Nothing can more negatively reduce the effectiveness of a team than a weak link or internal dissension. Each team member must be willing to give 110% to the team to facilitate team unity. When team members demonstrate their willingness to go beyond their assigned or perceived duties, it creates a contagious, participatory environment which promotes interoffice harmony. This internal harmony leads to a feeling of inner peace and a sense of pride that is readily sensed by colleagues and patients alike. If a team member senses that he or she is willing to go beyond the norm but one or more of the team is not doing his/her share, the internal peace phenomenon is disrupted and disharmony results. It is critical that each team member believe that every other team member cares about him or her as a person and respects his or her efforts to optimize teamwork.

Team members must ultimately feel empowered to make their own decisions about patient care as well as individual areas of responsibility relating to the practice. Once a staff member is trained and is qualified to act as an emissary of the practice, it is imperative that a feeling of support, guidance and confidence exists to affirm the special relationship that a busy practice demands. Creativity and spirit should be appreciated and acknowledged. Every team member seeks approval and recognition; therefore, words such as "Please" and "Thank You" should be regularly used expressions of communication. There are many ways to show appreciation to staff … but I believe the greatest expression of appreciation is to treat the team members as part of a family. Team members should be well compensated with as many perks as can be justified. They should be provided a clean, enjoyable environment in which to work, which should be free of bickering and petty gossip. Any new staff member can quickly surmise if the office setting is one of fairness and openness. Team leaders should want team members to contribute to, and enjoy the benefits of, a successful practice. A trusting, loyal staff does not "just" happen; rather, what happens if there is a "just" practice is a trusting, loyal staff. The stability of a contented staff is manifested in many ways. As of this writing, five members of our team each have in excess of 23 years service with our practice. The value of this longetivity of service is manifold, from not having to train new employees, to ultimate familiarity with our team concept. Many former patients who now bring their children or grandchildren to our practice have expressed loyalty to our practice as a result of the loyalty seen in our team members.

I have heard nightmares about practitioners letting go of trained, trusted employees because of gradual salary escalations or because pension plan contributions must be made due to federally mandated minimal time of service requirements. Practitioners are not oblivious to the fact that new employees can be recruited at much less salary, and eligibility for retirement benefits set at 2-5 years before funding occurs. However, this blatant disregard for team building flies in the face of fairness and completely undermines any credibility of the team leader. No member of any staff can profess allegiance to such a practice. Economics may dictate that employees be forced to work in such a practice, but their loyalty is compromised by such misguided attempts to deprive effective team members their due. We are, after all, brothers and sisters in the Human Race, and fairness and justice should be practice values paramount above all others.

One of our current team members, with more than 23 years in our practice, originally came to us as a result of a general house cleaning of staff by another local practitioner. This practitioner was purging his practice of employees who were approaching vesting eligibility in the corporate pension and profit sharing plan. This purge of staff members (I am reluctant to use the term "team" members because I believe you can't have a team without an effective team leader) by this practitioner turned out to be a godsend for our practice. This particular team member demonstrates to us daily the value of keeping someone who has bought into the team concept. One of her exceptional strengths is training new personnel, and her patience and experience are prized.

Employee turnover may not be just disruptive to your practice, but can also be very costly. Estimates of turnover costs, including lost productivity and new employee recruiting and training, range from $10,000-$40,000 per staff member, depending on his/her position.

A general business rule of thumb is that to replace an employee "costs" at least one times annual salary.

Staff Positions

1) Front Desk

The front desk is the portal to a practice. It is the first point of contact that a prospective patient has when making an appointment. Therefore, it is imperative that it be staffed with employees with outstanding people skills, a complete awareness of office protocol and positive, upbeat personalities. The front desk team members must excel at duties of a multiple nature, ranging from office greeter to receptionist, to bookkeeping, to appointment scheduling and chart filing, even to, in some cases, office manager. In many offices, handling insurance claims is also a primary responsibility, with some employing a part-timer, up to some employing as many as two fulltime staff members to handle this ever expanding practice headache. However many staff members work at the front desk, it is imperative that these diplomats who put the initial face on our practice, be presentable, well-groomed, constantly smiling, courteous and gracious. They should have excellent phone handling abilities and an overall awareness of office pace. They must be friendly, good listeners and still control any conversation so that they can also tend to the massive front desk duties. It is important that the front desk be amply staffed. Adequate monitoring by the team leader/leaders to verify that the front desk team members are properly representing the best interests of the practice is critical.

We have all experienced what we perceive as rude, insolent treatment by front desk personnel at professional offices. Such treatment has often influenced us to make a decision to take our business elsewhere even before we have actually seen the practitioner. In many instances, these "slights" will affect not only the practice image, but also its bottom line.

Some practitioners may be surprised if an assessment of their front desk were to be made by an independent analyst. One technique is espoused by a leading practice consultant who, as part of her services to her client, calls the office posing as a potential patient. She asks questions of the front desk staffer which allows her to assess the manner in which the call was handled. She evaluates courtesy, knowledge of the office, and the manner in which the patient's concerns were handled. Her assessments allow the team leader to shore up weak points in front desk team protocol, of which the practitioner may have been totally unaware.

Some front desk personnel have extroverted, friendly personalities but are, unfortunately, excessive talkers who perceive their primary front desk responsibility as being to entertain patients and parents.

Although this staff member is well liked by everyone, usually including the staff, there is a distinct possibility that such an employee is lacking in many of the qualities that are essential to being an effective front desk team member. Remember, to be effective, a front desk team member must be friendly, a good listener ... and still be able to control any conversation so that he/she can also tend to the massive front desk duties. Normally, these duties are so demanding that excessive talking will subjugate his/her responsibilities and another staff member will end up doing a disproportionate amount of the front desk work. There is a time and a place for everything, and even friendly, extroverted personalities must be kept in control.

Some practitioners may have what they perceive as a very skilled, protective front desk staffer who handles most situations without most issues ever reaching the team leader's desk. Sometimes it's handled on the phone by selecting which calls get through and which ones are to be called back. Sometimes it's responding to a patient's concern by attempting to reconcile any problem personally. Normally the staff member is only doing what he/she feels is "keeping the wolf from the door," and these protective actions are often appreciated by practitioners. However, such protective practices can add a layer between the practitioner, the practitioner's colleagues and patients. Remember the adage "The buck stops here." There are not many issues that should not be bounced off the practitioner to allow the decision to be made as to how each issue is to be handled.

A word regarding the subject of dishonest employees should probably be made at this time. This topic is never pleasant and all too often is considered something better swept under the carpet. It is sort of an enigma, a puzzling occurrence that always comes as a surprise and always by a trusted employee with access to practice funds. The very fact that the embezzler was trusted makes the loss a tragedy with dual implications. First is the loss of practice funds; secondly, and perhaps the most unsettling and shocking, the practice has lost a trusted employee. Never has an incident where a trusted employee embezzled funds ever been forgotten. If your faith in humanity is strong enough, you may forgive such an offense, but you will never forget. It is much more traumatic than a holdup or a burglary because embezzlement involves a breach of confidence.

We have been fortunate to have never experienced a dishonest employee, but the issue is out there and we are aware of several good practices that have had the misfortune to have been victimized.

There are guidelines established by experts who can explain that if you do such and such, your chances of being a victim of embezzlement are minimized. Always the foundational recommendation is to have a system of checks and balances in effect so that no one person has sole access to office books and office funds. They also recommend regular monitoring of office day sheets ... I can only add to these guidelines the following advice ... pay employees a just wage, provide them with a workplace that strives for fair and equitable standards and treat everyone like part of a family. It is not my intention to imply that if employees are trusted as family members and are well compensated, that embezzlement could never occur. Unfortunately, all of us are aware of more and more incidences of individuals stealing from their own families as drugs, gambling and greed are ever-increasing sociopathic concerns in our fast moving culture. I can only say that a fair wage, a just and equitable workplace with a familial atmosphere may not prevent embezzlement, but it certainly makes the act a more personal assault and perhaps less likely to occur.

Our Practice Office Manual specifically lists several offenses that we consider objectionable enough to warrant immediate dismissal:

- violation of confidential information
- embezzlement of funds, equipment or supplies
- fraudulent forgery
- improper use of drugs or alcohol
- conviction of a felonious charge

The guidelines are exacting and uncompromising. To date, I am gratified to report that the practice has never had to enforce any of these specific guidelines.

2) Clinical Floor

This critical position in most practices includes nurses, assistants, hygienists and technicians, and usually includes the team members with whom the practitioner works most closely on a direct basis. Most are highly trained, possess superior hand-eye coordination, are technically proficient in all phases of clinical treatment and are people persons who enjoy one-on-one contact with patients. Health services are one of the few professions where practitioners and team members actually touch patients. This implied trust agreement is a special privilege afforded our professions and we must be extremely respectful of it. All procedures performed on patients should be as pain-free as possible. Any techniques used while working on patients should be polished to the point that a patient's remembrance of any procedure performed includes the positive impression that every precaution was taken to diminish pain and every conceivable pleasantry was extended while the procedure was performed. Remember the adage "Do unto others as you would have them do unto you." The clinic floor is the perfect arena to practice this axiom on a regular basis and is a major component of successful practice building.

Where do these highly trained, clinic savvy team members come from? Most are graduates of university programs or licensed vocational schools, but some are recruited from newspaper ads and have previously related experience in another practice. Occasionally, resumes arrive in the mail from experienced staffers who have worked elsewhere and are new to the community. Others, though inexperienced, may impress a practitioner with their aptitudes, attitudes and work histories. It is worth remembering that significant time and investment is made in training a novice. Due diligence must be made before using this particular tact. Many practitioners also feel that psychological testing is of significant benefit when considering hiring any new staff member. Some practitioners are convinced that testing for aptitude should be a prerequisite when seeking a lab or clinical technician.

This may be an appropriate time to comment on what I feel is a very important consideration in hiring any employee into a practice. Because the team concept is paramount and any perception of favoritism is taboo in any practice, the employment of relatives or friends is not recommended. The hiring of friends or relatives is strongly discouraged as any occasion warranting reprimand or dismissal can be extremely stressful on both parties involved. The one certainty in the event such an unfortunate scenario ever occurs is weeping and hysterics and hurt feelings, not just from the disciplined employee but from family members and friends as well. It is far easier to address the issue, preempting any potential problem, by simply making it a non-issue by adopting an office policy stipulating that relatives and friends will not be employed. If there is one pearl that you take from reading this book, take particular heed of this recommendation.

3) Laboratory Technicians

Many practitioners have in-house labs for drawing blood, doing blood workups or, perhaps, pouring up dental models, making orthodontic appliances or any of countless other specialized duties. Usually these specialized duties are handled with minimal contact with patients and/ or parents and, in many instances, with other team members as well. Not only must lab techs be extremely talented, self-starters, and maintain a high level work ethic, they must also be amenable to the absence of person-to-person contact for long periods of time. Some practitioners feel that a special personality is called for and test for certain attributes when recruiting for this important team position. Psychological testing, as well as aptitude tests, is usually recommended.

4) Back Office Employees

Payroll – Some practitioners find it preferable to handle payroll themselves, often with software that makes this easier. Others find it preferable to have their spouses assume the duties of handling the practice payroll so that they become part of the practice staff with the duties performed at home, separate from the office setting. Others prefer that this duty be assigned to an office manager or front desk staffer. Yet others prefer to outsource payroll to a company specializing in handling office payrolls. There are many options available and individual preferences usually evolve over the years.

5) Consultants, Attorneys, Accountants, Bankers, Financial or Investment Consultants, Insurance Agents, etc.

Each of these practice overseers plays a different but integral role in the development and continued vitality and well-being of the practice. Some practitioners prefer to bring aboard family friends, fellow church members or seek recommendations from other practitioners. I personally favor discussing these very important decisions with other practitioners who have had previous experience with their choices and are willing to share their thoughts. Whatever your choice … closely monitor all relationships and be prepared to move the practice business dealings elsewhere if a reason to do so is perceived.

The selection of staff members is one of the most critical decisions a practitioner can make. No matter how diligent the investigatory attempts to determine that the applicant being reviewed meets the criteria that your practice calls for, it is still a win some – lose some proposition. By all means, personal and previous employment references must be checked and legitimate questions asked … a minimum of an initial and at least one follow-up interview should be made … and at least one interview by office team members is recommended. But still, in some instances, time is of the essence, or another office is also interviewing the same applicant and, after careful consideration, it is up to the team leader/leaders to make the ultimate decision rapidly, but with as much confidence as possible.

It is suggested that a minimum 90-day probationary period be set forth in the employment agreement, so that an ample time frame is allowed to determine the new employee's work ethic, attitude, ability to interact with patients and fellow team members and, most importantly, ability to adapt to the office philosophy of quality, courtesy and respect for everyone. It also allows time for the new employee to judge if this particular career path suits his/her objectives and satisfies his/her needs.

Sometimes the chemistry is just not right. Sometimes employees are slow to grasp the goal of teamwork. But every employee should be given every chance to adapt to the office protocol. Sometimes counseling may, in fact, be in order. Sometimes, even after experiencing the benefits of both patience and being provided every opportunity to adapt to the office protocol, an employee still is unable to perform at the level required. At this point, a decision must be made. Not every person is destined to work in the health professions, and it is not in everyone's best interest to continue to pursue something in which they are not qualified or in which adequate interest is not demonstrated. It is always preferable to address the issue sooner rather than later and in a constructive manner.

The SECOND Key – Enthusiastic, Effective Staff

- The stability that a happy, secure, hardworking team provides plays an integral part in the success of any practice.
- When team members demonstrate their willingness to go beyond their assigned or perceived duties, it creates a contagious, participatory environment which promotes interoffice harmony.
- This internal harmony leads to a feeling of inner peace and a sense of pride that is readily sensed by colleagues and patients alike.
- The words "please" and "thank you" go a long way to show respect and appreciation.
- There are many ways to show appreciation to staff but I believe that the one way that is most appreciated is to be treated as a part of a family.
- Team leaders should want staff members to contribute to, and enjoy the benefits of, a successful practice.
- A trusting, loyal staff, does not "just happen"; rather, what happens if there is a "just" practice is a trusting, loyal staff.
- The front desk is the portal to the practice and is the first point of contact that a prospective patient has with the practice.
- A front desk team member must be friendly, a good listener ... and still control any conversation so that he/she can also tend to the massive front desk duties.

- There are not many issues which should not be bounced off the practitioner to allow the decision to be made as to how each issue is to be handled.
- Basic guidelines ... pay employees a just wage, provide them with a workplace that strives for fair and equitable standards and treat everyone like part of a family.
- The clinic floor is the perfect arena to practice the axiom of "Do unto others as they would have done to them" which is a major component of successful practice building.
- Many practitioners feel that psychological testing, as well as aptitude, is of significant benefit when considering hiring any new staff member.
- All staff members do not necessarily have to be direct employees. Contracting and outsourcing can often provide attractive alternatives.
- The hiring of friends or relatives is strongly discouraged because any occasion warranting reprimand or dismissal will be extremely stressful on both parties involved.
- Not every person hired is destined to work in the health professions, and it is not in that person's best interest to continue to pursue something in which he/she is not qualified or in which adequate interest is not demonstrated. It is always preferable to address the issue sooner rather than later and in a constructive manner.

The THIRD Key
Practice Ethics

One dictionary definition of ethics is: "a system of moral principles or values; the rules or standards governing the conduct of the members of a profession; accepted principles of right and wrong."* A practitioner could translate these words as doing the right thing in terms of fairness, openness and morality. As your practice develops, you will make many decisions that reflect back directly on you, your family and your practice. If your desire is to have a rich life, not only monetarily, but mentally and physically as well, conducting your practice in an ethical manner is key. There can never be justification for deceit, misrepresentation, cheating patients or the government, or for that matter, any abuse of staff or of the doctor-patient relationship. Stress is self-induced! Each unfair, unjust action that we are responsible for adds a layer of stress. Some actions may skirt legalities, but are unethical, and we must make decisions focusing on the ethical value as well if we are to keep our conscience clear. We need to be able to comfort ourselves with the knowledge that what we did was the "right" thing to do.

* Ethics 4 Everyone, 2002 Performance Systems Corporation, E. Harvey, S. Airitam

In a previous chapter I mentioned a practitioner, obviously mindful of federally mandated minimum time of service requirements, who purged his practice of employees approaching vesting eligibility in his corporate pension and profit sharing plan. Apparently, that practitioner had tailored his Corporate Pension and Profit Sharing Plan documents so that an employee was required to be employed for two years to become eligible for pension and profit sharing benefits. Partial vestment over several more years would be required before full 100% vesting was realized. This arguably legal maneuver certainly resulted in enhanced short term profitability … but, in my judgment, it was not only unethical but a contemptible offense, inflicted on a blameless employee by a practitioner who skirted legalities for personal enrichment. A perverse abuse of the doctor-staff relationship of this type is fraught with potential peril to the practice's underpinnings. No practice can be successful when such a blatant disregard for fairness and justice exist.

It is too easy to rationalize doing something that we know is unethical because "everyone else is doing it" or because it is not illegal. Our practices should be like our word – above reproach. Each of us is accountable for what we do personally, and collectively as an organization. If we perceive that a professional organization to which we belong is doing something that is unethical, it is our responsibility to challenge any such activity. There is an old adage which seems to speak to this very issue … "Once you have seen the light, you can't hide in the dark!!"

It concerns me that our professions appear to be moving away from the standard of ethics that once was so rigorously pursued by our predecessors. The emphasis on money and material things is a powerfully addictive influence, and it has turned many a practitioner's focus from the pursuit of ethical standards. The tremendous pressures of debt repayment and the enveloping awareness that the practitioner, who has spent four to seven more years in school after college, lags significantly behind high school and college friends on the socio-economic scale, can influence decisions made in early stages of practice development. These early decisions may forever determine the type of practice that is established.

If we, as practitioners, are to merit the trust that we seek from our patients and the public in general, it is not only incumbent but critical that we maintain ethical practices. It is my judgment that when ethics are compromised, a gradual demoralization of the practice begins. Stress inducers are cumulative.

What are our moral values? If fairness and justice are not two of the cornerstones, we are on the wrong path. If your intention is to have a practice that you and your family can be proud of, one that is admired by your patients, your colleagues and by the staff that makes up your team, then living your life and conducting your practice according to ethical standards is the key. Every Key to a successful practice revolves around placing the highest value on the human being (not money or materials things) as the center point of the practice. If you pursue the things that will enrich your practice – justice, fairness, two-way respect, and upholding ethical standards, monetary rewards will find you as well.

Times are such now that our very culture is being challenged by a philosophy of "What's in it for me?" -- a philosophy brought about by excesses and lack of accountability which, in turn, accounts for the ever-widening gap between what is right and what will bring the biggest reward. This is also a time when practitioners entering the professions are experiencing the realities of monumental costs associated with opening a practice, of massive student-loan repayment debt, and of an awareness that former college classmates have moved to start their families and have progressed toward financial stability while practitioners attended graduate and post-graduate schooling. From this socio-economic awareness, as practitioners begin to establish their practices, they will make decisions in the short term that will define their practices as long as the practice exists. It is in this arena that decisions on philosophy of treatment, staff management, and marketing, as well as choices as to how the practice is conducted, are made. It is critical at this time that practitioners resist the inclinations to cut corners, to be less than honest with patients and insurance carriers, and to exploit the staff-doctor relationship relative to regulations, benefits and balance.

I can vividly recall, when I opened my practice doors over 35 years ago, a discussion with an older colleague about how things were going in my new practice, during which I reported that I had seen several new patient exams but that, unfortunately, nearly all were being placed on recall status. (At that time, conventional orthodontic treatment was generally deferred until eruption of all permanent teeth.) His well-intentioned advice to me was "to get some braces on those teeth ... get some money coming in." These were recommendations that I readily dismissed, but I could understand the temptation. Obviously, the suggestion was not for me to do something illegal, but the action, if intended solely to generate revenue and not for the benefit of the patient, was unethical. Just as extending a restoration onto another virgin dental surface, or referring certain questionable-need patients for an MRI or CT Scan to a company-owned imaging service, might not be illegal activities, such activities surely pose ethical questions.

It is incumbent on every practitioner to be aware of how our professions garnered the respect of the public we serve. We must be mindful of how this respect is ours to lose in the event that this special trust is not treated with the reverent respect it deserves. Our predecessors in the professions demonstrated selfless concerns for their patients ... by making house calls, working for fluoridation of community water supplies, promoting and demanding development of medicaments and materials specific to certain disease and illnesses. These selfless acts were not lost on the general public, who both trusted and respected these paragons of health care. Their trust set the stage as the Health Professions eventually came to enjoy the ultimate confidence of the general public.

This delicate bond between the patient and the practitioner is both fragile and tenuous and can only be maintained if the members of our professions conduct their practices in the most ethical manner. Remember, the high road is the only road if the professions are to survive in their current form. Every decision made in conducting a Practice should be just, fair and equitable. If decisions are made using those values as guidelines, stress will no longer be a concern. An ethical practice will flourish and long-term success will result.

THE THIRD KEY – PRACTICE ETHICS

- A successful practice is perceived by patients, by colleagues within the profession, by the staff and the team leaders as ethical, courteous, quality oriented and respectful of the patient-doctor relationship.
- If your desire is to have a rich life, not only monetarily but mentally and physically, as well, then conducting your practice in an ethical manner is key.
- Some actions may skirt legalities, but are unethical, and we must make decisions focusing on the ethical value if we are to keep our conscience clear and find comfort knowing that what we did was the "right" thing to do.
- Each of us is accountable for what we do personally, and collectively as an organization. As a member of a professional organization, we have the responsibility to challenge any activity by that organization that we perceive to be unethical.
- If we practitioners are to merit the trust that we seek from our patients and the public, it is not only incumbent but critical that we maintain ethical practices.
- The bond of respect that patients have for practitioners is both fragile and tenuous and can only be maintained by members of the professions conducting their practices in the most ethical manner.
- If you pursue the things that will enrich your practice --justice, fairness, two-way respect, and upholding ethical standards, -- monetary rewards will find you as well.

The FOURTH Key
Pursuit of Excellence

The pursuit of excellence should be a major objective of every practitioner. I can remember when I first opened my office doors, that my principal practice building conviction was that if you do quality work, it would follow that people would seek you out. I am no longer so naïve, -- I have gradually become aware of the many other tangible and intangible factors that go into building a successful practice. However, I still feel that the pursuit of excellence is one tenet in the successful practice that remains a constant. I can tell you about many practitioners who maintained high standards of quality of treatment yet did not have, what I would consider to be, successful practices. Yet I know of no successful practices, by my explicit definition, where the pursuit of excellence is not a persistent, sought after objective.

From the very first day we open our practice doors, we must assume responsibility for, and gain personal gratification from, making our patients happy. We must demonstrate a fundamental commitment to excellence that patients, staff, and colleagues perceive as a constant, ongoing standard of treatment. This is the genesis from which all successful practices must spring.

The pursuit of excellence begins with confidence in your abilities to successfully manage whatever problems are presented by the patients who come into your practice. If you graduate from professional school and you do not feel that you have a confident grasp on all the intrinsic factors associated with treating patients at the highest possible levels, do not hesitate to seek additional training prior to starting your practice. Depending on your personal perspective, you may know a seasoned practitioner with whom you can associate until he/she retires and you can take over ... or perhaps specialty school ... or a residency of some sort ... or even enlistment as a practitioner in the armed services to refine your skills. Whatever your choice, be certain that you are confident in your capabilities to provide quality treatment before committing to the pursuit of excellence.

A good friend of mine, Dr. Gary Inman, after graduation from post-graduate training and in the process of opening a practice in a smaller town approximately 50 miles from our practice location, asked if he could work two days a week in our office until his practice became sustainable. His request stressed that he wanted to "learn the right way to straighten teeth." This mutually beneficial association took place for almost two years and developed into a friendship that has blossomed over the past 25 years. I could easily recommend this approach since it seemed to be a viable means to allow his integration into a busy practice routine and, at the same time, allowed our developing practice the benefit of his many talents. I am hopeful that he gained as much from the associate relationship as I did, including the expansion of my knowledge base concerning the value of having team diversity.

Once we are confident in our capabilities to provide quality treatment, the next step in the pursuit of excellence is to recruit a team that shares your focus on structure, inter-action with people and a sense of ethics. Some employees have started at one position and moved or gravitated to another as the need arose. The primary consideration is to obtain the type of people who embody the practice's pursuit of excellence philosophy. Our practice seeks continual feedback in exit surveys about the performance of team members, as well as perspectives on how patients perceive their time in treatment. (A copy of our exit survey is included in the glossary of this book.) Some practitioners suggest periodic surveys be disseminated at appropriate times so that an assessment of how patients and/or parents perceive their practices can be analyzed. This simple, straight-forward survey request serves a dual purpose. First, it allows an assessment of how a practice is perceived by providing an anonymous vehicle for patients and/or their parents to use to express their impressions as to the strengths and weaknesses of that practice. Second, the patient and/or parent is made aware that the practitioner is interested in their perceptions by giving them the opportunity to comment anonymously. Upon completion of treatment, we routinely request that an exit survey (anonymous) be filled out and mailed back to our office in a pre-stamped, self-addressed envelope. This keeps us aware of patient perceptions of our practice. Thankfully, negative comments are rare (most deal with waiting room comfort, or suggesting Saturday hours, or different office music, etc.) Obviously, some comments require immediate action and others are to be dismissed. By far the most frequent comments that have been expressed in a written form are comments favorable to the staff and the quality of treatment received. This is a major consideration in our pursuit of excellence. The comments about our undersized reception room are addressed in the new office building that our younger associates planned. On the other hand, consensus on office music can never be reached, (and, frankly, I'm not sure I could live with it, even if it was.) When the practice first opened 36 years ago, I worked Saturday mornings. I was attempting to develop a practice, and it seemed like one good way of attracting patients. However, I found that the patients attracted by the Saturday morning hours, disproportionately missed more appointments than others, were disproportionately slow payers and oftentimes seem to be people looking to take advantage of the new kid on the block. After nine years of Saturday morning appointments, and with a great amount of trepidation, I decided to discontinue Saturday hours. I feared that the move would seriously hamper practice growth. But the practice continued to grow as before and both team members and I were elated not to face Saturday morning appointments again.

Once we are confident in our capabilities to provide quality treatment and once we have assembled what we consider to be a conscientious team who represents the type of practice that we strive for, it behooves us to utilize internal marketing to publicize this commitment to quality treatment to both patients and colleagues. In an orthodontic setting, there can be no greater joy to the parents of a child, who have made a significant sacrifice of money and time by placing their child's care in your hands, than to receive high quality before-and-after photos of the facial and dental changes associated with comprehensive treatment. It also makes sense to accompany these photos with a personalized letter, personally signed by the practitioner and staff members. These photos and accompanying letter are virtually assured of being shared with family members, relatives, bridge groups, church groups, school mates, neighbors and friends everywhere. What greater recommendation of your pursuit of excellence could be conveyed to the community? This one example of internal marketing of your practice is worth far more than the largest ad in the phone book. There are certainly similar internal marketing concepts available in other disciplines aside from orthodontics. It can be accomplished with photos every time that restorative work is done on a patient's dental needs or by physicians sending a before and after x-ray scan print of a fractured bone; or by a personalized note following the resolution of an illness, along with countless other personalized correspondence with patients following treatment in your practice. Everyone would like to know that our concerns in the patients we care for are genuine, and the more treatment is perceived as valued by our patients, the more the images of our profession and our individual practices benefit.

The pursuit of excellence requires adherence to a simple set of guidelines -- always strive to do every procedure, research every decision, and prepare for every possible scenario to the best of your abilities.

Even after you have completed the necessary schooling, passed whatever tests are required for licensure, and eventually opened the doors to your practice, you have just begun to enter the realm of Practice Management. No courses in the Health Science curriculum can adequately prepare you for dealing with people on matters of patient service and satisfaction. Do not be deluded into thinking that the success of your practice is synchronal with the grades you achieved in Biochemistry and Gross Anatomy. All that is behind you now, and you must be aware that the primary determinant of practice success is how you deal with people. If you set your practice goals to be a people practice, concentrating on service, respect and fairness, your practice will be grounded on the rudimentary principles of practice success. These basic objectives are much more meaningful than obtaining all A's in graduate school, or purchasing the most prominent ad in the telephone directory, or building the largest and most elegant professional building in the community.

Extraordinary service may be extended to patients in a variety of ways, and practitioners should be aware that the same courtesies that impress them as consumers should be considered when establishing an office policy. Treating patients with dignity, respect and a sincere smile should be standard, established practice protocol.

How a practice reflects honesty, integrity, dependability, cheerfulness and morality are strong indicators of the type of practice being conducted and the type of service patients can anticipate. If the team leader/leaders convey these attributes (both in and out of the office setting), it can be readily assumed that the team members within the practice will also reflect similar values.

Be ever mindful that the pursuit of excellence does not end with the quality of treatment provided. A practitioner can produce consistently exceptional quality treatment with superior treatment mechanics and still not obtain, by my explicit definition, a successful practice. A successful practice emanates from the pursuit of excellence that is a committed effort to provide quality treatment in a practice dedicated to patient service and satisfaction. The successful practice treats patients, colleagues, team members and the general public with respect and honesty, and does so in a sincere, consistent, cheerful manner. The successful practice puts an emphasis on values and service. Build your practice on this foundation and success will follow.

The FOURTH Key – Pursuit of Excellence

- Quality of treatment and the pursuit of excellence should be major concerns of every practitioner.
- I know of no successful practices, by my explicit definition, where the pursuit of excellence is not a persistent, sought after objective.
- We must demonstrate a fundamental commitment to excellence that patients, staff and colleagues perceive as a constant, ongoing standard of treatment. This is the genesis from which all successful practices must spring.
- The pursuit of excellence begins with confidence in your abilities to successfully manage whatever clinical problems are presented by patients who come into your practice.
- Once we are confident in our capabilities to provide quality treatment, the next step in the pursuit of excellence is to recruit a team that shares your focus on structure, interaction with people and a sense of ethics.
- Once we are confident in our capabilities to provide quality treatment and have assembled a conscientious team which represents the type of practice we strive for, it behooves us to utilize internal marketing to proclaim this commitment to quality treatment to patients and colleagues alike.
- If you set your practice goals to be a people practice, concentrating on service, respect and fairness, your practice will be grounded on the rudimentary principles of practice success.

- A successful practice emanates from the pursuit of excellence that is a committed effort to provide quality treatment in a practice dedicated to patient service and satisfaction.
- The successful practice puts an emphasis on values and service.

The FIFTH Key
Positive Practice Image

This positive practice image (as perceived by our patients, our colleagues, and the general public) is not an easy undertaking, nor something that can be earned overnight. It is the culmination of many instances of people talking to other people about things that have impressed them. People are impressed with many things, but their impressions form the practice image. Images can be positive or negative and it bears pointing out that, according to psychologists who study images, negative images are much more likely to be shared with other people than are positive images. We've all heard the old adage that "do something good and one person knows, do something bad and 14 people know."

An incident comes to mind of a practitioner who, while in a discussion with a patient and her mother, became so incensed when the patient's cell phone rang and the patient did not end the conversation quickly enough to suit him, walked away from the situation and refused to return.

We must not work only to obtain a favorable image but work, at least as hard, to avoid unfavorable images of our practices. This one incident had the potential to significantly undermine the many positive efforts that had been made on a daily basis to enhance that practice's image. How could this situation have been handled more appropriately? Some practitioners have signs at the reception desk asking that all cell phones be turned off while in the office setting. Or, the practitioner might have stated "If you want to take that call, I will have to return to your needs when I can work you in ...". Whatever it takes to avoid a confrontation in a no-win situation should be the primary objective when situations such as this present themselves.

I submit to you that most consumers are not aware of how to assess quality of treatment but make determinations of which practices they choose to do business with based almost exclusively on hearsay and recommendations. Some practitioners may have the good fortune to have the only game in town, but for the rest of us, image is everything!

A positive image is accomplished not only through quality treatment, but also by being friendly, by treating people fairly and by being considerate of their needs. It is also critical that each patient and parent be greeted with a smile and that an effort be made to make them feel comfortable in the practice. The practice is made up of many individuals, all of whom form a confluence to one common image of the practice – either favorable or unfavorable. To this extent, one must never let himself or herself become complacent. Each member of the practice team must perform his or her duties with pride, with a smile and with the satisfaction that the very best he or she can do will be done every time. The effective team leader must orchestrate these staff efforts so that dedicated, committed team members are performing their duties properly and that unfavorable, unpropitious habits are not introduced into practice protocol. If these basic principles are consistently demonstrated by staff members and by the team leader or leaders, there is no way that practice can have an unfavorable image.

Each of us has unfavorable images of some business or health-care provider in whose place of business we experienced what we considered to be a "slight." Perhaps this unfavorable experience was the result of a curt remark by a front desk staffer in response to a question ... or ambivalence to the fact that our scheduled appointment was 20 minutes ago with no explanation or apology offered … or even a condescending, flip dismissal of a concern that we've expressed. Most "slights" are non-intentional and may be simple miscommunications. But once our mindset experiences a negative perception, changing that perception is very difficult. In many instances, it is not the team leader but a staff member who is responsible for this "slight." It is not reasonable to expect staff members who have not bought into a team concept to project favorable positive perspectives. The team leader may sign the paychecks, but no staff member should ever make the mistake of assuming that their primary objective is keeping the team leader satisfied. It is incumbent on all members of a practice to understand that they work for, and are indirectly paid by, our patients. Therefore, they have personal responsibility for providing extraordinary service to patients. Inattentive staff members can do as much harm to practice development as attentive staff members can help practice development. Courtesy and respect are imperative character traits associated with positive images and successful practices.

In the course of everyday conversation, many of us are aware of countless reports by disgruntled friends who have languished in waiting rooms for an hour or more past their scheduled appointment time. Many of these incidents occurred without any explanation or justification by staff members for such an outrageous disregard for the patient's time, and the cavalier, callous disdain for the contract of trust that should exist between the practitioner and the patient. Signs should be placed in several locations within the office, including on the reception counter, advising patients that anyone waiting longer than 15 minutes past their scheduled appointment time to please contact the receptionist. If for some rare reason, a patient is kept waiting more than 15 minutes past their scheduled appointment time, 1) an apology should be made, 2) an explanation of what caused the problem should be given, and 3) an assurance should be given that the patient will be seen as quickly as possible once the reason for the delay is resolved. This implied contract of trust is a fragile, capricious bond that is subject to mutation at every offense, either real or imagined. Therefore, every practitioner should be appreciative of a busy practice, but work to assure that they and their staff are doing the elemental things necessary to keep it that way.

This is probably a good time to discuss the first impression conveyed to a patient upon entering an office and being greeted by a sliding glass window separating the waiting room from the practice reception area. It is my perspective that such a sliding glass window serves as a barricade between the practice and the patient. It presents an "ours versus yours" appearance. I find it extremely difficult to project a friendly, welcoming ambience to patients entering an office when a sliding glass partition is the first contact presented. It can be perceived as a negative precursor of what to expect. It is my judgment that, as practitioners who seek the public trust and, who encourage and recruit new patients into our practices, it is incumbent upon us to sacrifice the semi-privacy of a sliding glass barricade to the welcome a smiling, friendly front desk team can convey. This does not mean that surgery should be visible from the reception room, but all people feel more comfortable when talking to a human voice rather than listening to a voice prompter, and would rather observe the inner workings of a busy practice front desk team as they go about conducting their everyday workload, as opposed to feeling as an outsider on the wrong side of a glass partition.

One of the longest enduring trademarks of health care practices is the sliding glass partition. Other changes, some dealing with efficiency and others with practicality, have been rapidly assimilated and it is my judgment that this particular idiosyncrasy will soon be a thing of the past. One of the primary goals of every business, whether a health care provider, a corner restaurant, or a multi-million dollar corporation, should be to maintain a positive image.

If there ever was an objective to be pursued by a practice in its quest to be successful, it is to the attainment of a positive image by colleagues, patients, staff and the general public. Practices able to achieve a favorable image do so by hard work, meticulous attention to treating people with respect, giving extraordinary service, and providing what patients perceive to be excellence in quality of treatment. It is obvious to any consumer that image can make or break a business. Those with favorable images must work to sustain this image and those with less than favorable images must work much harder in an attempt to upgrade this perception. A negative image, once labeled, cannot be changed by placing an ad in the newspaper or phone directory proclaiming the practice's virtues ... or by lowering fees to entice a shopping clientele into the office. The only manner in which a negative image can be changed is by addressing the issues that resulted in the development of the unfavorable image. Sometimes, it may mean terminating the employment of a staff member who has not bought into the team concept. Sometimes the unfavorable image can be traced to actions or character traits of the practice leader/leaders and, if that is the case, upgrading the practice image is even more of a formidable task. I have heard of practitioners leaving a site where the practice image was considered negative by colleagues and patients, and starting over in another city or state.

Though it would be impossible to quantify a relationship between a practice's image and that practice's success, it is not difficult to imagine the correlation. Every practitioner and every team member must be attuned to the critical need for a positive practice image. Every effort must be made to assure that the perception the general public has regarding the practice is a favorable one.

THE FIFTH KEY – POSITIVE PRACTICE IMAGE

- Negative images are much more likely to be shared with other people than positive images.
- We must not work just to obtain a favorable image but work at least as hard to avoid unfavorable images of our practices.
- Most consumers are not aware of how to access quality of treatment and make determinations of which practices they choose to do business with that are based almost exclusively on hearsay and recommendations.
- Each member of the practice team must perform his or her duties with pride, with a smile and with the satisfaction that the very best he or she can do, will be done every time.
- It is incumbent on all members of a practice to understand that they work for, and are paid indirectly by, our patients.
- If at all possible, sliding glass partitions should be avoided as a separator between the reception desk and the reception room. This will serve to convey a more welcoming, friendly practice ambience.
- Though it would be impossible to quantify a relationship of a practice image and practice success, it is not difficult to imagine the correlation.
- One of the primary goals of every business, whether a health care provider, a corner restaurant, or a multimillion-dollar corporation, should be to maintain a positive image.

The SIXTH Key
Cutting Edge Technology

Technology in every practice should be maintained at cutting edge levels, in the forefront of what is available in the industry. There is a fine line between premature, unconstrained jumping into products and procedures that have not been adequately tested in the open market, and well investigated utilization of the most advanced, up-to-date materials and techniques known and accepted within the profession. Each of us can recall being pressured to write prescriptions for a drug that we felt was inadequately tested … or purchasing, after being persuaded by a magazine ad or article, an expensive tool or product only to find out that what we were previously using worked as well or better in our hands. Physicians are quick to recall the legacy of "Thalidomide", the once perceived "miracle drug" for treating morning sickness, which eventually was found to have caused severe birth defects in many cases when taken by pregnant women. Dentists still routinely are seeing severely discolored teeth caused by patients taking mega doses of wide spectrum antibiotics (usually tetracyclines) in early childhood during permanent tooth development. Many orthodontists recall the trepidation associated when removing ceramic brackets which, when first marketed, formed a chemical bond to tooth enamel when the brackets were placed on teeth. Incidences of fractured teeth, enamel fractures, gouges in veneer facings and crowns all were reported to have occasionally occurred when those brackets were removed. These ceramic brackets (chemical bonding, as compared to the current mechanical bonding) were marketed to the public before being adequately field tested, and, because of their instantaneous popularity, put orthodontists under immense pressure to add them as an elective to their armamentarium.

But for every drug or procedure that can be portrayed as having a negative legacy, there are countless others which have proven to be everything from life enhancing to life saving. We must never be satisfied with the status quo. Better products and appliances are constantly evolving and allowing for improved treatment of patients. The key appears to be the characteristic of being well researched and standing the test of time.

I can recall my astonishment in learning that an elderly dental practitioner in our community had lost a thumb, resulting from his routinely holding an x-ray film in his patient's mouth rather than have the patient hold the film or using a sterilizable filmholder. The high kilo voltage machines used in the past required much longer exposure time than current models, and practitioners who routinely subjected themselves to this prolonged exposure were placing themselves at great risk. Thankfully, this was a rare occurrence, but succinctly emphasizes the need for an awareness of the dangers of materials and machines with which we work. This practitioner was only attempting to obtain better quality radiographs in the most expeditious manner. Even materials and machines which can be considered safe have to be treated with respect and a full comprehension of any dangers involved in their usage.

It is imperative to have an awareness of what is available in the marketplace for our professional needs. Keeping informed and staying abreast of changes is critical to maximizing professional standards and assuring that state-of-the-art patient care is always the primary consideration of any practice. Regular attendance at continuing education courses and seminars should be planned into all schedules. Professional journals and periodicals should be read and discussed with colleagues to maximize the benefits to be garnered from your reading efforts. I am fully supportive of Study Clubs formed by practitioners involved in similar disciplines that meet on a regular basis with assigned reports on certain subject matters presented by members to the entire membership. The showing of interesting cases, successes and failures, with comprehensive records, should be a scheduled agenda item at the meeting, with members presenting on a rotational basis. New procedures, instruments, techniques, practice pearls, etc., should be shared among the group and a free exchange of information encouraged. Study clubs should be inclusive, but limited to no more than 10-12 members in order to gain maximal benefits and so a frequent rotation for presenting articles and cases is allowed each member. Meetings sites should be rotated and, probably, be held on a quarterly basis. Members should be selected based upon their sense of responsibility, ethics and quality of treatment.

Studying the literature, attending continuing education courses and active participation in professional study clubs are effective assurances that you are being exposed to updated technology. Utilization is then the choice of each practitioner, but every practice striving to be successful must be computerized, using maximally effective sterilization techniques, and state of the art equipment, such as digital cameras, radiology equipment and instruments. There are many among us who remember not too long ago, prior to the advent of latex gloves, and when the most common method of instrument "sterilization" was cold sterilization (Zephryn Chloride). Thankfully, those days are over and our practices, professions and the public we serve are the better for it and our practices have evolved into being part of the greatest health care system anywhere. We are indeed fortunate, but should not become complacent. We must keep up with advances in technology as they become known to us, lest we be left behind in the rapidly developing changes within each of our chosen disciplines.

There are many practitioners crying out for less governmental regulation of our practices and demanding that our professional associations work toward influencing that objective. But be ever mindful that if government regulators (through its OSHA arm) had not mandated that all practitioners be required to wear disposable latex or non-latex gloves when treating patients, there would be practitioners still performing procedures on patients without gloves. There would be practitioners still using Zephryn Chloride cold sterilization rather than autoclaves, and there would still be practitioners without lead-lined walls in rooms where x-rays are taken. We all can certainly understand the critical nature of disposable gloves and the use of autoclaves as barriers to the spread of disease, and we must all, likewise, understand that not all regulations are personal hardships forced on practitioners. Without regulators to force the non-compliers and the practitioners lacking awareness of ... or disregarding ... cutting edge technology, and requiring compliance with regulations benefiting and protecting patients and practitioners alike, our professions would collapse into chaos. Some regulations, when initially proposed, are misdirected and, in some cases, unnecessary. However, most of these are normally discontinued or altered after a while since the element of time has a way of sorting out the necessary versus the non-necessary.

Many of us recall the fateful tragedy that befell the profession of dentistry in the early 1990's when a Florida dentist was linked to the transmission of the AIDS virus to six of his patients. You may also recall the epidemic of fear that swept the country at the time and the knee-jerk reaction of some state legislatures to the issue. In the state of Kentucky, legislation was passed that mandated three <u>annual</u> hours of required H.I.V. Continuing Education to all dentists and dental hygienists in the state. This legislation was enacted despite the fact that this one case in Florida was the only case where a patient-dentist relationship was proven. This mandated annual C.E. requirement was enacted in 1990. This legislation applied only to dentists and dental hygienists and not to physicians.

The catastrophic nature of the AIDS virus and its potentially devastating effect on an innocent community was a major concern of the general public, and regulations were put into place by the Kentucky State Legislature in a direct strike at the state dental profession.

Fortunately, the mollifying effects of time and the lack of other incidences eased the public's fears of a dental link to transmission of the virus and the regulation was eventually modified to a more practical requirement when in 2001, it was changed to a more reasonable standard of one three-hour C.E. requirement every ten years.

Again though, the need for regulations to protect the public, practitioners and practitioners' staff is obvious. We are, above all, dedicated to the safety of our patients, and, understandably, regulations are a necessary part of that safety net.

The SIXTH Key – Cutting Edge Technology

- Technology in every practice should be maintained at cutting edge levels, in the forefront of what is available in the industry.
- We must never be satisfied with the status quo -- better products and appliances are constantly evolving, allowing for improved treatment of patients.
- Keeping informed and staying abreast of changes are critical to maximizing professional standards and assuring that state-of-the-art patient care is always the primary consideration of any practice.
- Studying the literature, attending continuing education courses and active participation in professional study clubs are effective assurances that you are being exposed to updated technology.
- We must keep up with advances in technology, lest we be left behind in the rapidly developing changes within each of our chosen disciplines.
- There is a necessary need for considered and reasonable governmental regulations within our practices.
- Without regulators to force the non-compliers and the practitioners lacking awareness of ... or disregarding ... cutting edge technology or forcing compliance with regulations benefiting and protecting patients, staff members and practitioners alike, our professions would collapse into chaos.

The SEVENTH Key
Working Environment

The environment that makes up a practice includes more than the outer and inner walls; countless other factors must be taken into consideration when evaluating our daily work site. Common sense dictates that each of us prefers to work in an environment that is fun, uplifting and satisfying. Bright colors and smiles should be plentiful. Pleasant background music and appropriate dress is a welcome rendering to our senses. Cleanliness is imperative!!! Comfortable seating and work stations are mandatory. There is never a reason for anger or obscenities. Pleasantries between staff and patients, and between each other, should be an ongoing occurrence. ("Pleasantries", meaning cheerful small talk, such as a comment expressing awareness and appreciation of a new hairstyle, dress, etc. or an inquiry about how school is going or what travel plans are being considered.) Products, instruments and furnishings should be treated with respect. Appreciation for a sterile field is incumbent on us all and we have the responsibility to honor the trust that patients extend to us. Anything that can be recycled should be recycled.

(The subject of recycling braces is quite controversial,* and we have never used recycled braces, but I have no problem with it as long as the patient and parent are advised, given a choice, and, if the choice is made to use recycled braces, the savings are passed on to them.)

A sense of harmony should prevail. Order and organization should permeate the entire work site whether the office is empty or full. Respect for each other and each other's feelings is a must. A sense of quality and pride go hand in hand, as one necessarily flows into the other.

Each of us is aware of practitioners who, for one reason or another, have favorites on their staff who receive special privileges and benefits unavailable to other staff members. In rare instances, a sexual relationship may be involved; in others, perhaps just a naïve unawareness that staff members are generally aware of almost everything that happens in an office setting. Body language, small perks, and indications of partiality all are dead giveaways that can cause staff members to assume a sense of unfairness and bias. Nothing can be more detrimental to a team concept. There must never be any perception, valid or simply suspected, that a special relationship exists for one staff member that disrupts team unity.

The team leader is responsible for compiling an office policy manual that very specifically spells out the policies, protocol and regulations of the practice. This manual should be inclusive and deal with all subjects, ranging from parking, sick days and vacations, cosmetics, insurance and any other issue relating to work and workplace concerns ... extending all the way to felonies. The manual should mandate a code of conduct and corresponding penalties for failure to comply. All rules and regulations should be fair and administered to all in an equitable manner. A copy of our office policy manual, which is updated annually and which was in effect when I retired in 2006, is provided in the Glossary of this book. It

* There have been newspaper accounts of practitioners using recycled braces costing a fraction of the original retail price. Even though companies that sell recycled braces report a high level of quality control, some practitioners are concerned that machined tolerances and specifications for the original product may be compromised following usage, removal and sterilization prior to re-use.

is meant as a frame of reference only and should be considered as such. A copy of our sexual or environmental harassment manual, which spells out what our practice considers a fair and appropriate guide to what is allowed and not allowed, is also listed in the Glossary. Please do not underestimate the significance of having a printed manual addressing such issues. It allows for a more comfortable internal working relationship for all concerned, staff and team leaders, alike. One of our team members, after signing the sexual harassment manual, asked, "Does this mean that we can't tell dirty jokes anymore?" Of course it doesn't, as long as everyone is comfortable with the jokes, but if someone is offended and requests that joke telling be discontinued in his/her presence, that request will be respectfully honored and adhered to.

If an office has all the above characteristics, the likelihood of its being a successful practice is overwhelming.

Perhaps this is the proper time to discuss interoffice communication between team members. It is my judgment that discussion between staff and each other, if in the presence of patients or parents, should either include the patient and/or parent in the conversation or is better left unsaid. In fact, we encourage discussion between team members and patients and discourage small talk between team members when patients are present. We stress including the patient in all conversations and encourage friendly banter back and forth between the team leader, team members and patients. We want patients to feel comfortable, welcome and included. We want team members to consider the workplace as a place of business but, also, a place where the words "patients" and "friends" are synonymous.

The team members' response to their everyday working experience is predicated on how they perceive their working environment. If they perceive their colleagues as being respectful of each other, aware that each team member is willing to give 110% to their practice, and, feel that they are treated fairly and equitably by the team leader, they will do everything in their power to be an integral part of such an organization. They will demonstrate this positive outlook consistently and with confidence that they are part of a team doing great things for people and for themselves.

I am a firm believer in a favorable attitude and its effect on others that come into contact with this phenomenon. If a team member is pleasant, cheerful and engaging, it stands to reason that any patient who comes into contact with that team member will be influenced similarly. Contrast that scenario with one in which the staff member is curt, unpleasant and repelling or just simply has a bad attitude. As a team leader, which staff member would you rather have represent your practice? And remember, these experiences contribute piecemeal to our practice image.

I can tell you with certainty which experience the patient would rather have. And not only will this experience be impressed indelibly upon the patient's concept of your practice, you may not even have had the occasion to meet with the patient before this image of your practice was formed.

And now, let's go a step further ... to discuss what criteria should be emphasized when considering potential employees. It is my judgment that attitude is one of the most important traits to be evaluated when making decisions about potential future team members. Granted, it is difficult to get a feel for attitude in one meeting, and that's why at least one follow-up meeting is suggested along with an interview session with team members only. We then advise a 90-day trial period to evaluate attitude and aptitude, before welcoming the employee into permanent team member status. Once you have determined that a new team member has a favorable attitude, it is critical that he or she be continuously exposed to a fair and just working environment to keep it that way.

The SEVENTH Key – Working Environment

- Common sense dictates that each of us prefers to work in an environment that is fun, uplifting and satisfying.
- Order and organization should permeate the entire work site whether the office is empty or full.
- Discussion between team members and each other, if in the presence of patients or parents, should include the patient and/or parent in the conversation or is better left unsaid.
- Discussion between team members and patients is always encouraged, and small talk between team members is discouraged unless the patient is included in the conversation.
- The team members' response to their everyday working experience is predicated upon how they perceive their working environment.
- There must never be any perception, valid or simply suspected, that a special relationship exists for any one staff member that disrupts team unity.
- All rules and regulations should be fair and administered to all in an equitable manner.
- The team leader is responsible for compiling an office policy manual that very specifically spells out the policies, procedures and regulations of the practice.
- Attitude is one of the most important traits to be evaluated when making a decision about potential future team members.

The EIGHTH Key
Essential and Non-Essential Expenses

The subject of expenses is always perplexing, and one that cannot be specifically delineated into "do this" and "don't do that". Every practitioner has to decide for himself or herself what are justifiable expenses and what are extravagant and unjustifiable. The first basic tenet about practicing a profession is to equip the staff members with the knowledge and instruments needed to be successful. The second basic tenet mandates that any expenses necessary to allow you to provide outstanding service to your patients are to be considered essential expenses. These two categories of expenses are non-debatable and, once identified as such, must be budgeted for. Any expenses other than these two categories are debatable and each practitioner must make decisions relative to what he or she feels appropriately represents the practice's best interests. For example, is giving away a toothbrush to every patient a justifiable expense? Or coffee in the reception area? Does using only the highest quality materials fit your practice needs or would you prefer to charge less and use less expensive materials? Each practitioner, after satisfying the two basic tenets mentioned above, is on his/her own when deciding what other expenses are justifiable. Some expenses are considered fixed expenses and represent a relatively constant monthly practice liability. Even these fixed expenses (rent/mortgage payments, gas and electric, taxes, insurance, etc.) are controlled in a large part by the team leader/leaders' perception of practice needs. Generally speaking, the larger and more grandiose the practice facility, the higher the fixed expenses portion of your monthly budget.

Some practitioners consider expenses as something expended to secure a benefit or bring about a specific result and are influenced by their perception of "what the competition is doing." Advertising and office design are two examples of responses to concerns about competition. Some practitioners aspire to have the most appealing, attractive office in the community and feel that any expenditure toward that goal is a justifiable expense. Some practitioners believe that advertising expenses are not only justifiable but necessary to bring patients into the practice. There is no right or wrong answer as to justifiable expenses. I can only relate to you a reflection that I have previously touched upon ... In my judgment, patients perceive a practice as being successful not by the amount of advertising the practice does, nor by the splendor of the facility it is housed in, but rather by how the team and team leaders relate to each other and to patients in their care.

The practitioner must be aware of commonly accepted guidelines that break down ratios of expected expenses relative to revenue; i.e., percentage for staff salaries, percentage for rent, etc. These guidelines are not to be considered cast in stone but do offer a comparative analysis of how your practice compares to other practices when comparing fixed and non-fixed expenses as a percentage of revenue.

There are several aspects about my education (or lack of) that I have learned to live with, but, to this day, still regret. Number one is that I never took a typing course in school. The high school I attended, based on Entrance Exam Test scores, divided the students into three classifications: Scientific, Business and General. If you scored high enough on the entrance exam, you were placed in the Scientific curriculum and the core of subjects taught to you related to math and science. Typing was an elective and, for some reason (over 50 years ago), there were very few in our classification who elected to take it. Thus, still today, I am a hunt-and-peck, very limited typist. My second regret is that I never took a business course in high school or college and felt overwhelmed when I attempted to obtain an MBA at the University of Chicago. I was working as a Chemist at Sinclair Research Labs in South Chicago at the time. I passed a test that allowed me into the University of Chicago night school MBA Program. But, one semester later and after studying at least as hard as I ever did for any science course, a "C" in Accounting and a "D" in Economics sent me scurrying in another direction – to Dental School at the University of Louisville. After a couple of years in the Service during the Vietnam War, I completed my post-graduate training in Orthodontics at Northwestern University Dental School. I eventually opened an orthodontic practice in Louisville but felt I knew virtually nothing about how to run a business.

I was fortunate to have joined an Orthodontic Study Club which consisted of 12-15 orthodontists from all over the state of Kentucky. Several of the members shared the same accountant, and I joined the list shortly after opening the practice. Gerald Psimer has been our practice accountant for the past 34 years and has graciously served as a sounding board whenever a situation occurred that warranted a knowledge of business. If he didn't know the answer, he would advise me whom to contact to resolve my dilemma. He has been a confidant, an advisor and a friend.

When opening a practice, some practitioners may not have developed a relationship with an accountant that they feel comfortable consulting with when making business decisions. But if your circumstance was in any way similar to mine, you may feel the need to explore contracting with a business manager to make sure that someone is paying attention to the business side of the business. It is not at all unthinkable that a practice could flounder or even fail because of poor business skills.

I would recommend that each practitioner study and read about management and leadership as much as possible. There are many good books, tapes and seminars available that can go a long way toward educating a new professional about a practical understanding of the business side of a profession. Cornerstone Leadership Institute (www.cornerstoneleadership.com) has many good books and tapes that present excellent overviews of management and leadership. I recommend them highly.

Consultants and Newsletters – Essential or Non-Essential?

It is with a great deal of trepidation that I enter into this arena of which I have always had serious misgivings. As our practice evolved over the years, we have subscribed to several prominent practice advisory newsletters, and I feel they do have a place in following legal and legislative changes involving practice management. These newsletters kept us aware of current litigation proceedings, changes in legislation that affected practices and businesses, ways to maximize office efficiencies and, in many cases, controlling costs (albeit it appears, in most cases, at the expense of staff.) The primary function of a practice advisory newsletter is to enlighten the practitioner as to the legal alternatives available relative to maximizing profitability. Some of the typical "strategies" recommended by some newsletters on how to maximize earnings by controlling staff costs include designing or re-designing existing retirement plans to limit eligibility, and by adding a provision that allows the practitioners to use his/her age to provide maximum plan contribution allocations for himself/herself, while limiting younger employee contribution allocations. Other newsletter recommendations include maximizing part-time employee staffing while keeping hours worked below the levels required for eligibility for fringe benefits and retirement plan allocations. Paying employees on an hourly basis rather than salary basis and only when the practitioner is in the office is another suggestion. An additional "strategy" is to increase staff benefits rather than salary increases, thereby allowing the practice to avoid payroll taxes and retirement plan contributions funding on the fringe benefits provided. (Actually, this last strategy may be the only one to provide a symbiotic benefit to both the practitioner and the employee since increasing benefits rather than increasing salary does allow the employee to avoid paying taxes on these benefits.)

I once again point out that each of these strategies is concerned primarily with controlling staff labor costs and maximizing profitability, not with team building or practice building. I am not a proponent of building short-term practice profits at the expense of under-rewarding team members. The choice is each practitioner's to make ... When dealing with staff concerns, is the primary focus geared to building a successful practice or to maximize profitability? Are the two mutually exclusive? Does one feed into the other? My concern is that short-term focus on maximizing practice profitability can tend to destroy long-term practice team effectiveness. As I have indicated earlier in this book, I firmly believe it should be the team leader's goal to take comfort and pride that his/her team is reimbursed at competitive salaries with as many perks as can be rationalized. This doesn't mean that attention to costs not be heeded, but team members have bills to pay, children to raise and a need to feel pride in their employment. If you consider staff loyalty and dedication to be a necessary practice mainstay, nothing stimulates appreciation for team leadership more than a feeling that all are part of a family with the common purpose of making the practice as successful as possible. Please allow me to reiterate ... A trusting, loyal staff does not "just" happen; rather, what happens if there is a "just" practice is a trusting, loyal staff. My perspective remains the same – our practice pays the staff well, provides excellent benefits, has fees in the mid-to-upper echelon in our community, takes our share of Medicaid cases as a community service, and, instead of giving out country hams at Christmas, donates the approximate cost of an orthodontic case to a Louisville Dental Society designated charity every year in the honor of our referring dentists. Yet, in spite of this, or perhaps because of it, our practice has been very successful in terms of profitability and community image and retention of long term team members who excel at the team concept. You decide which avenue appeals to you the most!

On the other hand, I must admit to a shortcoming in our practice protocol that was addressed and corrected by a Consultant in one visit to our office. It used to be typical practice philosophy that when patients were seen in our office, the maximum treatment that could be performed was performed on each patient at each visit. It was my belief, at the time, that these maximum treatment mechanics were justified, even if it extended into the next scheduled appointment, because it allowed the patients to complete their orthodontic treatment earlier. Because we had adequate staffing and super team "esprit d'corps", we would eventually catch up, but it did result in reception room backup at times. Thanks to the recommendation of a Practice Consultant, this protocol was abandoned and more rigid time allotments were established and adhered to. Once we changed to better defined timed slots for patients (i.e., 15 minute, 30 minute, 60 minute, or 90 minute appointments) any patient who showed up late or had extensive repairs which required more time than allotted, was stabilized and reappointed to a more appropriate time slot. This allowed for a less harried staff, a more harmonious office flow, and, most importantly, it did not result in patients who showed up on time for their appointments having to wait while we finished maximal procedures on someone whose work requirements extended past their slotted time.

This is just one of many office procedures that we changed after visiting a good friend of mine, Dr. Jud Knight, in Lexington, Kentucky. Jud was ecstatic about what he considered major policy changes in his office protocol after engaging the services of a consultant, Ms. Jackie Thurman, from League City, Texas. He invited me to visit his office to observe and decide for myself. I have always admired Dr. Knight as a clinician and a person, and I eagerly accepted the invitation. It turns out that Ms. Thurman was the former office manager of a leading clinician in Texas and had decided to branch out into practice consulting. She initially impressed me when I phoned her, and during the course of the conversation, told me that she limited her services to one practitioner in any given community. At a time when one's livelihood depends on the number of clients one has, it was refreshing that she felt it important that no conflict of interest nor even a hint of impropriety could ever be a source of concern to her clients. We scheduled a visit, and all of us, team leaders and team members, were immensely impressed with her in-depth analysis and her straight-forward assessments and recommendations. To make a long story short, we decided to pursue most of her recommendations dealing with scheduling, billing, collections and taking on additional personnel. Initially, some of the changes suggested by Ms. Thurman were met with skepticism by team members and team leaders, alike. When you have been doing something along similar lines for 30 plus years (and bear in mind that five team members have been with us for 23 plus years), the threat of change, when things have been perceived to have been going well, presents concerns. In essence, we had to make choices ... Does because we have been doing something well for 30 plus years make it the best way to do things ... or are we willing to scrap a major portion of our office protocol to allow the recommendations of an acknowledged expert in the field after a fair evaluation of our practice? As we gradually worked our way into the recommended changes, numerous team meetings were held and, over a period of time, we began to see the many benefits of the changes. I now feel strongly that the changes in our office protocol brought about by Ms. Thurman were significant, meaningful, and beneficial, not only to the team, but to patients, as well.

The team has now taken ownership of Ms. Thurman's recommendations. Her follow-up reports are carefully studied as we strive to give full exposure to areas that need shoring up. We have elected to maintain slight digressions from some suggestions, but in general, we have bought the Full Monty.

One of the major tenets that she espoused was the need for making the most accurate assessment possible of treatment time and/or case difficulty when discussing that subject matter with patients or clients. She emphasized that patients would rather have an accurate assessment of total treatment time, so that they can have a realistic anticipation of what to expect, rather than be expecting one thing and experiencing another. She reports that some practitioners tend to underestimate the difficulty of the case or the treatment time involved in order to be able to quote a lower fee for the procedure. This serves to prevent the fee from jumping to a higher level (thus minimizing "sticker shock") by underestimating the difficulty of treating that particular case, but often results in the patient feeling misled when the quoted time frame arrives and treatment is not yet completed. The most accurate assessment possible of treatment time and case difficulty at the consultation presentation, along with discussion of any recourse if treatment is finished early or later, is strongly stressed by Ms. Thurman.

I am now a devotee of practice consultants, particularly Ms. Thurman, and recommend that all practitioners engage a consultant to look at their practices with a critical eye. I have come to realize that doing something the same way for a number of years, even though the process is comfortable in your hands, does not necessarily make it the best way. There is a place for consultants in a practice, no matter your particular discipline.

The EIGHTH Key – Essential and Non-Essential Expenses

- Every practitioner has to decide for himself or herself what are justifiable expenses and what are extravagant and unjustifiable expenses.
- The first basic tenet about practicing a profession is to equip the staff members with the knowledge and instruments to be successful.
- The second basic tenet mandates that any expenses that are necessary to allow you and your team to provide outstanding services to your patients are to be considered essential expenses.
- Any expenses other than these two categories are debatable and each practitioner must make decisions relative to what he/she feels appropriately represents the practice's best interests.
- You may feel the need to explore contracting with a business manager to make sure that someone is paying attention to the business side of the practice.
- It is not unthinkable that a practice could flounder or even fail because of poor business skills.
- Most practice advisory newsletters deal with current litigation proceedings, changes in legislation that affect practices, ways to maximize office efficiencies and, in many cases, controlling costs (usually at the expense of staff).
- The practitioner must decide – Is the primary focus when dealing with staff concerns geared to building a successful practice or to maximize profitability?

- Short-term focus on maximizing practice profitability can tend to destroy long-term practice team effectiveness.

- If you consider staff loyalty and dedication to be a necessary practice mainstay, nothing stimulates appreciation for team leadership more than a feeling that all are part of a family with the common purpose of making the practice as successful as possible.

- Patients want the most accurate assessment possible of total treatment time so they can know what to expect, rather than be expecting one thing and experiencing another.

- Doing something the same way for a number of years, even though the process is comfortable in your hands, does not necessarily make it the best way.

- There is a place for Consultants in a practice, no matter your particular discipline.

The NINTH Key
Marketing Your Practice

Previous chapters have touched on marketing, both internally and externally, and yet the subject matter merits a more comprehensive discussion. There are numerous marketing techniques, and practice consultants can best describe to you some internal marketing concepts which have proven most effective for the various disciplines; i.e., sending out Before and After Treatment photos to patients, etc., in orthodontics. Different disciplines, when comparing effective marketing practices, require different levels of marketing as well as different types of marketing. That is to say, that the practice of law has become much more dependent on advertising than say, the practice of accounting. Advertising is only one arrow in the quiver of marketing, but it is indeed a major player. At a time when the pharmaceutical industry spends more on advertising than on Research and Development, it is only fitting that some additional light be directed to this comparatively recent phenomenon that has completely changed the dynamics of the practitioner's concept of marketing.

It was as recently as 1975 when the U. S. Congress passed legislation giving the Federal Trade Commission new powers to set industry-wide rules of conduct and to seek civil penalties against "expressive violators." At that time, the FTC began an antitrust suit against the American Medical Association that enjoined other professional groups under the same umbrella. The suit charged that the AMA ban on physician advertising discouraged competition and unfairly disadvantaged consumers. After years of legal battling, in 1982 the suit was ultimately resolved in favor of the Federal Trade Commission and the ban on physician advertising was lifted. The rest is history...

Billboards now scream out for the attention of the consumer. A trip through the yellow pages in any urban telephone directory features a multitude of ads proclaiming the benefits of selecting one practice over another. The ads are getting larger and more pretentious. All are designed to catch the eye and influence the decision of the consumer. Obviously, advertising must have some effectiveness to be able to justify the level of budget share that it has attracted. Advertising is expensive, and it is not guaranteed!

Depending on your point of view, advertising either offers the opportunity to highlight the nuances and benefits of your practice, or it places practitioners in a situation where they must decide to either become a public media advertiser or depend on internal marketing alone to promote their practices. Although all professional practices – law, medical, dental, veterinary, accounting, etc. – have many similarities due to their structure and being as an essential provider of services to the public, each is unique in its dependence on a referral basis. To one group of professionals, advertising can be considered an essential component of their marketing effort, while in others it is a minor consideration. Again, the professions of law and accounting are contrasted.

Whether advertising is or is not a critical component of marketing, it allows a practitioner to promote his/her practice by means of an exchange of currency for exposure.

This straight-forward purchasing of exposure has some special advantages. It allows for a relatively new practitioner to enter the arena without having to go through the hoops of traditional practice building.

It also allows bypassing dependence on the development of a referral base. But because of the significant expense of advertising, it must also have a proportionate level of effectiveness. There are more than a few practitioners in the Health Professions who have decided to carve out a slot in their budget to buy into the exposure for currency gambit.

Why is it, then, that the majority of practitioners in the Health Professions still are hesitant to start a major advertising campaign? Is it something other than the expense involved? Obviously, the answers are only conjecture ... however, some may rationalize that practitioners, both old school and new school, are reluctant to dim the patina of their chosen profession, that they hold in such high regard, by engaging in what they perceive to be something that detracts from the professionalism of their profession. Perhaps these practitioners have sensed the public lack of trust of advertisers in general. When the general public is subjected to the tawdry, distasteful, unrestrained claims that they are constantly bombarded with from phone book ads, billboards and TV/radio infomercials, it is quite possible that some lumping of all advertisers into one classification takes place.

Remember, the fundamental relationship between the professions and their patients is one based on trust! How does the general public rate the level of trust when asked to rank various professions and occupations on their perception of honesty and ethics? Public Perception of Honesty and Ethics, 2003-04 Gallup Poll, as published in the Winter Edition, Vol. 71, #4, Journal of the American College of Dentists, vividly points out the different levels of trust that the public experiences when compelled to interact with different professions and occupations.

Table 2. Public Perception of Honesty and Ethics, 2003-04 Gallup Poll

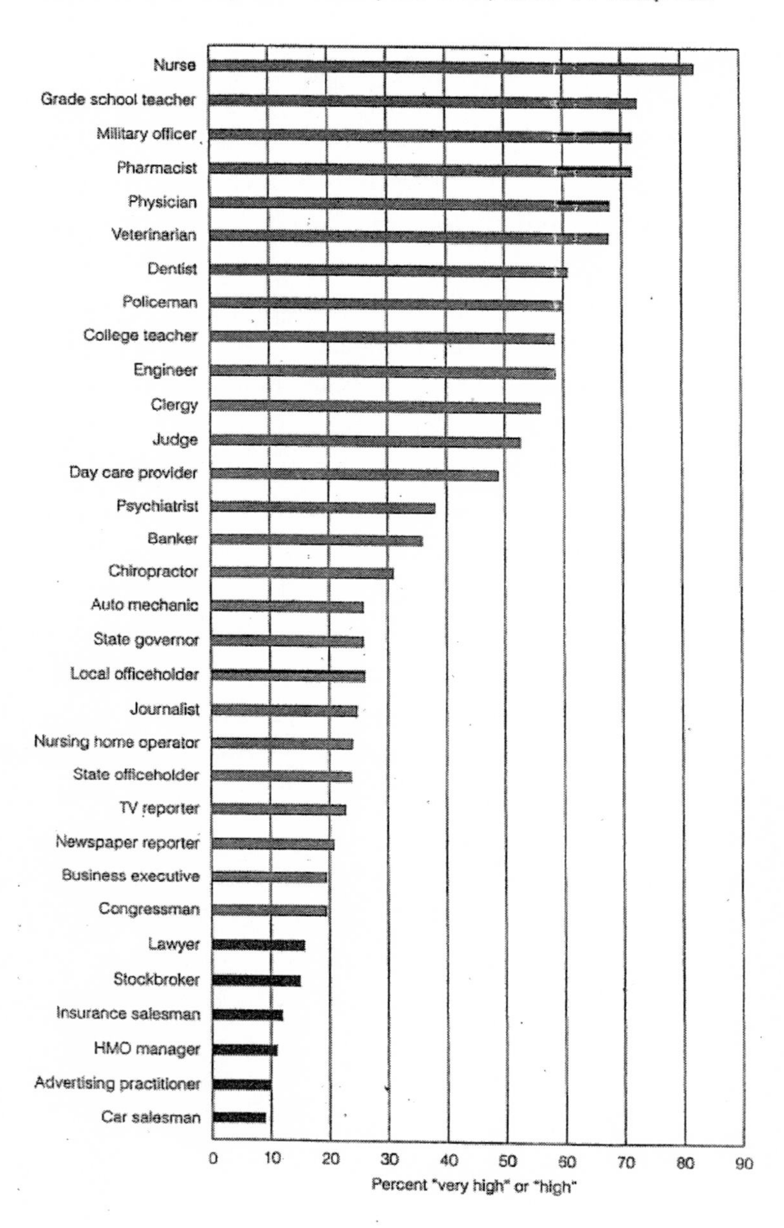

There are many interesting observations to be made, and conclusions to be drawn, which can lead to multiple hypotheses about why a particular profession or occupation is ranked where it is. In fact, such interpretations could probably be sufficient subject matter for another book.

The ranking of one category, though, is of particular interest to this specific section of this book. Does it surprise you to see "Advertising Practitioners" ranked where they are on the scale dealing with perception of honesty and ethics? The poll points out the number of respondents perceiving the honesty and ethics of advertising practitioners as "very high or high" was second to fewest, just above car salesmen, when ranking various professions. There is no doubting the veracity and prestige of the Gallup Poll, but can you believe that its polling in this instance is an accurate assessment of the general public's opinion? What is the rationale that the public draws from when making these kinds of judgments?

Advertising by professionals may now be legal but many of the claims made in the ads are virtually self-aggrandizement. The public in general has become very skeptical of this form of self-promotion. This lack of trust, however, doesn't mean that advertising is not effective. The basic criteria for determining whether to advertise or not advertise will always be money. And as long as those practitioners who advertise feel that as a result of advertising they are bringing more money into the practice than what advertising costs, they will continue to advertise.

Of course, it is both unfair and inappropriate to assume that all practitioners who advertise are self-aggrandizing. All of us are aware of competent, community-serving professionals who have elected to cast their lot with the advertising market. In a declining market share environment, it is tempting to revert to whatever is necessary in an effort to entice patients to the office door. My major concern, however, is with the public's perception of what defines a profession and what delineates a profession from a trade. Here is a listing of characteristics that were used in describing the word "profession" at the American Dental Association Managed Care Conference in Chicago, July

1995: high standards, knowledge, authority, power and privilege, promises (to place rights of patients above that of organization) code of ethics, and social organization. How does advertising relate to these characteristics?

I personally would rather think of my fellow practitioners in the profession as colleagues, not competitors, and am keenly aware that our predecessors have labored long and hard to make the profession what it is. It is only ours to give away.

Whatever your thoughts may be toward advertising, it is absolutely critical that you develop internal marketing within your practice, constantly searching for ways to improve what you can do to promote your practice from within. The literature is replete with suggestions about internal marketing from practice consultants, advisory newsletters, etc. Working to enhance your practice image is certainly effective marketing, along with the other suggestions previously mentioned when discussing other Keys.

The NINTH Key – Marketing Your Practice

- Different disciplines require different levels of marketing as well as different types of marketing. Advertising is only one form of marketing.
- In 1975, the Federal Trade Commission began an antitrust suit against the American Medical Association that enjoined other professional groups under the same umbrella. The suit charged that AMA ban on physician advertising discouraged competition and unfairly disadvantaged consumers. In 1982, the suit was ultimately resolved in favor of the FTC and the ban on physician advertising was lifted.
- Advertising allows a practitioner to promote his/her practice by means of an exchange of currency for exposure.
- Depending on your point of view, advertising either offers the opportunity for exposure to highlight the nuances and benefits of your practice, or it places practitioners in a situation where they must decide to either become a public media advertiser or depend on internal marketing alone to promote their practices.
- The majority of Health Profession practitioners do little advertising. Is it because of reluctance to engage in something that they perceive as detracting from the professionalism of their profession?
- According to the 2003-2004 Gallup Poll Public Perception of Honesty and Ethics, the general public does not perceive the honesty and ethics of Advertising Practitioners as "very high or high" when compared to a ranking with other professions.

- My major concern, relative to advertising, is with the public's perception of what defines a profession and what delineates a profession from a trade.

- It is preferable to think of our fellow practitioners in the profession as colleagues, not competitors.

- It is absolutely critical that you develop internal marketing within your profession, no matter what your feelings toward advertising.

The TENTH Key
"Ego" – Don't get the Big Head

Definition of ego from Andrew Cohen* - "Ego is the one and only obstacle to enlightenment. Ego is pride. Ego is arrogant self-importance. Ego is the deeply mechanical and profoundly compulsive need to always see the personal self as being separate from others, separate from the world, separate from the universe. Ego is a love-denying obsession with separation, narcissism and self concern."

This well-thought-out perspective on ego, defined by Andrew Cohen, is unmistakable in its meaning. To have love, to have enlightenment, we must strive to control our ego. As practitioners, it is easy to fall into the trap of exaggerated self-importance as we complete our education and move into the world of the professional. At that moment, the aura of being something special is there for the taking. We have worked hard, accomplished a major objective in life goals, attained the cultural level where respect has been secured with the potential to earn income such that we should never have to want for anything of a practical nature. We can hire and fire at our discretion

* Excerpted from "Living Enlightenment" by Andrew Cohen (Moksha Press, 2002)

and mingle with the movers and shakers of our community. We have much to be thankful for, and yet, it is quite facile to let ourselves be ensnared into mistakenly believing that we are superior to the general populace. There is a clear and distinct risk of an exaggerated sense of self-importance.

During our training and schooling, each of us has striven to excel ... to demonstrate superior ability as we competed against other students for recognition of our accomplishments and our abilities. Yet, once we achieve the goal of becoming the professional we aspired to be, we must then step back and reflect on what we really have. We are one of a few who resides in a country that allows each of us the right to an education, ... one of a few with the underpinning systems in place to allow us to attend school rather than have to work to support a family, ...and one of a few who was born at the right time in history to allow us and our generation the benefits of what our predecessors have established for us in the evolution of our profession to what it is now.

Every day, in our busy offices, we have people who present themselves to us, seeking our expertise and depending on us to provide answers to their questions and resolutions to their problems. We have staff members impressed with our knowledge and abilities as we give them direction and sign their paychecks. To patients, clients and staff members, we, as professionals, can take on the appearance of a "knight in shining armor."

Once the professional assumes the mantel of leadership and takes on the responsibility of being the professional, the battle with ego and exaggerated self-importance must be won. It is a never-ending battle, but one whose successful resolution is critical to being an effective team leader. There is no better indication of how successful a practice has become than by the respect a team leader conveys to the team, colleagues, patients and the general public. Whereas, a practitioner is a practitioner once the office doors are opened, the successful practitioner who is able to control ego is one who realizes that respect is a <u>two-way</u> street.

The effective team leader/leaders demand respect by being respectful of every person with which they come into contact. This same deferential esteem should be extended to patients, parents, staff members, vendors, janitors ... to everyone to the same degree respect would be conveyed to any colleague or to the President of a University or, for that matter, to the President of the United States. Respect is earned by showing respect for others. If you want respect, you must first earn it ... Look people in the eye, focus on what they are saying, be sincere in your interest in people ... and you are fulfilling your part of the two-way street called RESPECT.

The image of arrogant, haughty practitioners who show disrespect for their client or patient base because of their financial circumstance, race, creed, gender or sexual preference, affects the entire profession. These same practitioners may be active in their churches, but express disdain and contempt for minorities and the less fortunate. I assure you that the words these practitioners so eloquently use in their prayers have no meaning when contrasted as to how they treat the least among us. Theirs is a balancing act that has no foundation. "Love thy neighbor as thy self." This simple statement, if exercised, keeps ego in check and the focus on what it takes to make a practice successful.

Practitioners, know who you are! Control ego and direct your practices to be ones of respect for everyone and everything. Set your sights on doing the right things and for the right reasons.

THE TENTH KEY – "EGO" – DON'T GET THE BIG HEAD

- To have love, to have enlightenment, we must strive to control our ego.
- After attainment of professional status, there is a clear and distinct risk of an exaggerated sense of self-importance.
- To patients, clients, and staff members, we as professionals can take on the appearance of a "Knight in shining armor."
- There is no better indication of how successful a practice has become than by the respect a team leader conveys to the team, colleagues, patients and the general public.
- The successful practitioner who is able to control ego is one who realizes that respect is a <u>two-way</u> street.
- "Love thy neighbor as thy self" is a simple statement that, if exercised, keeps ego in check and the focus on what it takes to make a practice successful.

The Ten Keys to a successful practice presented in this book do not constitute a "magic pill" that, when taken, will simplify your life, reduce stress and guarantee that your practice is successful, and that your passage to heaven is assured. However, if serious consideration is given collectively to each subject matter discussed, a basic framework for a successful practice is assured. Remember that a successful practice is a perception by patients, by colleagues within the profession, by the staff and the team leaders that the practice is ethical, courteous, quality oriented and respectful of the patient-doctor relationship. If you do that, you can't go wrong!

EPILOGUE

In writing a book about The Practitioner's Credo: 10 Keys to a Successful Professional Practice and my judgments about ethics and how they relate to a successful practice, I feel it both relevant and necessary to advise any reader that my membership in the American Association of Orthodontists has been revoked by the Board of Directors of the Association. If the author is to be taken seriously when commenting on ethics and how they relate to the profession he chooses to write about, any digression from the Association Line warranting revocation of membership needs to be addressed.

After spending over 34 years in the profession that I have truly loved, orthodontics has provided me with more blessings than I have ever deserved, friends and colleagues sharing common bonds, and literally thousands of smiling, happy faces that I see daily as I come and go within our community.

I have been privileged to serve in leadership positions both within dentistry and orthodontics. I was elected to serve as President of the Louisville Dental Society and as President of the Kentucky Dental Association. I served six years as a Delegate to the American Dental Association, both contributing to, and challenging Association policies. I am a member of both honorary dental fraternities – the American College of Dentists and the International College of Dentists – and have served on and chaired numerous committees within local, constituent and national organizations.

I served a two-term presidency of the Kentucky Orthodontic Association, and as President of the Southern Association of Orthodontists (the region representing the 11 Southern states – Alabama, Florida, Georgia, Kentucky, part of Louisiana, Mississippi, North Carolina, South Carolina, Tennessee, West Virginia, Virginia.) I served a six-year term on the Membership, Ethics and Judicial Concerns Council of the American Association of Orthodontics, three of which I served as Chairman. I also served as Alternate Delegate to the House of Delegates of AAO for several years. I am a Board Certified Diplomate of the American Board of Orthodontics and have been a member of the College of Diplomates of the American Board of Orthodontics for many years.

I must also point out that I served as Chairman of the Kentucky Dental Association Political Action Committee (KDA-PAC) for several years because, at one time, I was convinced of the merits of such an organization. I am now convinced otherwise. In 2003, I received my annual ADA dues statement of $841.00 with a qualifier notice that $64.21 was allocable to lobbying activities. About the same time, my AAO dues statement of $865.00 arrived with a notice that $16.94 of the dues was for lobbying expenses. The qualifiers explained that the amounts allocable to lobbying activities were not a deductible expense. For 32 years I had systematically responded with a check for the full amount within the week, never questioning the amount of dues or any assessment that was mandated by the respective House of Delegates. This time, I sent checks to both organizations, but withheld the amount stipulated as being for lobbying activities.

I now have some serious misgivings with buying "access" to legislators and, so, I wrote letters to both the ADA and AAO Board of Directors (copies of letters in the Glossary), expressing my opposition to the process. I explained that I felt lobbying expenses and contributions to legislators should be limited to a voluntary basis only. I offered to pay the full dues to both the American Dental Association and the American Association of Orthodontists if my point of view was published in the monthly Association newsletter circulated to the general membership. I suggested a point-counterpoint forum where both sides of the issue be presented and responses encouraged. The American Dental Association printed my statement in the form of a letter to the editor, and I immediately paid the dues in entirety. The American Association of Orthodontists refused to provide a forum for my concerns, and a letter, signed by all members of the Board of Directors, was sent August 24, 2003 notifying me that partial payment of dues was unacceptable. My check in the amount of $848.26 was returned uncashed.

In November, 2003 I requested the mailing list of all orthodontists in the United States and Canada from the AAO. I was notified on December 4, 2003 that my membership in AAO was revoked for non payment of dues. On December 9, 2003 I received a letter notifying me that my request for the mailing address list was denied due to my membership being revoked for nonpayment of dues, and with the additional statement that even if I still held membership in the AAO, the nature and scope of my mailing would not be considered to be within the scope of the AAO policy of selling mailing labels.

A copy of the letter that I had intended to send out to the full AAO membership also appears in the Glossary for your edification.

• •

So, here is my position … as of December 31, 2005 I am now a retired orthodontist. My membership in the American Association of Orthodontists has been revoked for refusing to pay the $16.94 portion of my dues that is deemed dedicated to lobbying expenses. I have always believed in standing up for what I believe in and will continue to do so. I am humbled and honored that you have chosen to read this offering to the professional. I hope and pray that this small expression of my love for the profession will be of benefit to you in some small way, no matter how small.

It is fitting to offer a special thanks to my wife, Joyce, who provided all the typing, proofreading and much of the motivation for this book, as well as working to help put me through both graduate and post-graduate training. She has been to our practice what the sun is to the earth; to my son, Chris, who has taught me the pleasure of having blood in the practice and who has done so much to develop the practice and carry it forward; and to Marybeth Averill, who, as a patient, paid us a high compliment when she confided that she uses our office as an example of a successful company when discussing company policies. She is the

Vice President of Employee and Organizational Development for a large corporation in Nashville, Tennessee. During one of her office visits I explained that I was in the process of writing a book about professionalism and ethics, and had several chapters completed. I asked if she would consider reading them and critiquing what I had to say. She was truly a God-send. I can never thank her enough for her patience, her contributions, her guidance and her commitment to helping me find my way. One of her initial suggestions, when I was talking to her about chapter topics, was to be sure to write about "Ego – don't get the big head." Writing about ego was the easy part, but I never would have considered the idea if it wasn't for her. Later, after reading what I had written at the time, she made several other suggestions that helped immensely with keeping my focus on the task at hand. I stand eternally grateful for her much appreciated beneficence.

I also owe a huge debt of gratitude to Jeff Stamper, a personal friend, occasional golf-mate and attorney nonpareil. He has been instrumental in helping me through many endeavors, and perhaps the most challenging for both of us … bringing this book to fruition. In his college years, Jeff minored in English, and his editing skills have been invaluable. His sage counsel, good humor, and suggestions were also timely, dependable and appreciated.

And, lastly, I want to express my appreciation to the Team Members … both Louisville and Bardstown … who have made "our" practice what it is. Their willingness to expend tireless energies, boundless enthusiasm and unimaginable l'esprit du coeur, always with an unwavering smile, is a testament to both their character and their intellect. These teammates have bought into the concept of team, and no one appreciates their loyalty more than the team leaders and the patients, that together, we serve.

Appendix A

PERSONNEL POLICIES AND PROTOCOL

For the offices of

Mattingly & Howell Orthodontics, P.S.C.

2317 Stony Brook Drive
Louisville, Kentucky 40220
(as of July, 2006)

208 N. Second Street
Bardstown, Kentucky 40004

A GUIDE FOR OUR STAFF

AS OF 2005

NOTE: **The policies in this manual are subject to change at anytime but will be used as guidelines for purposes of normal office protocol.**

Table of Contents

EMPLOYMENT APPLICATION

Please provide the following information on the separate sheet of paper provided for that purpose:

- Name, Address, Phone Number, Social Security Number, Position Sought and Previous Related Training.
- Previous occupations in past five years.
- Please list several character references other than family.
- Do you have any limitations to prolonged length of service?
- Please list expected starting salary and fringe benefits.

On the reverse side of your application page, put any additional information you may wish to provide. Is there any question you would like to ask about the office or the position you are seeking?

BRIEF SUMMARY OF OFFICE POLICY

SALARY - Based on previous experience and average salaries within the dental profession in the Jefferson County area. No automatic pay raises but a minimum of an annual review of daily work record, salary and expectations of duties and responsibilities.

BENEFITS - Pension Plan, Life and Disability Insurance, Uniform Allowance, Vacation, Sick Days, 125 Cafeteria Plan availability and 401K Fund Matching Retirement Plan.

VACATIONS - Paid vacations after 12 months of employment are based on the number of hours worked per week. A comprehensive discussion of vacation, vacation eligibility and formula for determining such is discussed in detail in body of text.

HOLIDAYS - New Years Day, Memorial Day, Fourth of July, Labor Day, Thanksgiving, Christmas and additional days which may be selected at the discretion of Mattingly & Howell Orthodontics, P.S.C.

PERSONAL DAYS - No time off is allotted for personal days but time out of the office may be charged against credited Sick Days or Vacation Time.

SICK DAYS - Sick Days are provided at the rate of five per year for full-time team members and prorated accordingly for part-time team members. Those who work four days will receive four days and those working three will receive three days, based on the same formula as vacation day determination.

LEAVE OF ABSENCE - Special circumstances will dictate individual handling of an event, but a position can only be protected in accordance with Family Leave Act Provisions.

CONDITIONAL EMPLOYMENT PERIOD - Three months from first day of duty.

WORKING HOURS - 7:00 am – 6:00 pm daily with one hour for lunch (current lunch hour) 12:45 pm – 1:45 pm.

PERFORMANCE REVIEW - At least annually or per the request of individual team member.

OTHER POLICIES - Personal telephone calls, personal appearance, performance of duties in our absence, medical and dental appointments, housekeeping, parking, outside employment, personal orthodontic care, smoking, discipline, and dismissal are explained in complete detail in body of text.

THE POWER OF TEAM

Our orthodontic practice is a people practice. The success of the practice depends on many things; the results of completed cases, the reputation among our peers and the public, the trust and confidence of our patients and their parents and the feeling from within ourselves that we have done the very best that we can do for our patients and have done it in a manner that reflects personal pride in a sense of accomplishment. It is the patient who determines the number of employees in our practice, just as it is the patient who determines the ultimate success of any practice. As long as we have a sufficient patient load, we have the luxury of dictating office hours, specific work days, and even appointment scheduling of during-school visits on a rotational basis. Every attempt should be made to make the patients and their parents comfortable and feeling that their interests are our primary concern. Each team member in this practice has specific responsibilities that he/she is obligated to perform. Each team member is also expected to perform his/her duties with pride, with a smile and with reflection that the very best they can do will be done every time.

GOALS – A FAVORABLE IMAGE

The establishment of a good reputation is not an easy undertaking, nor is it something that can be earned overnight. It is the result of many instances of people talking with other people about things that have impressed them. People are impressed with different things, but their impressions form our image. The formation of a good image has to be considered a primary goal of our practice. It is accomplished by being friendly, by treating people fairly and being considerate of their needs. It is also necessary that we maintain a positive attitude as well as being able to successfully treat orthodontic problems. While the building of a favorable image requires many positive actions over a prolonged period of time, this favorable image must be maintained on a daily basis or it becomes tarnished and suspect. To this extent, we must never let ourselves become complacent or at ease with ourselves or our duties. Our ongoing goal is the maintenance of a positive image with the public and with our peers.

COMMUNICATION

Effective intra-office communication among personnel is imperative. One hand must know what the other is doing or chaos can result. The lines of communication must be open at all times and utilized to facilitate the running of an orderly, synchronized practice. Regular team staff meetings which include all team members are held periodically (currently every sixth week from 11:00am to 1:00pm) and will rotate between the Bardstown and Louisville office sites. Every sixth week (three weeks after combination meeting), a team meeting specific to the Louisville and Bardstown offices is held at those particular sites. Each team member will chair the meeting on a rotational basis, and the minutes will be posted and reviewed at the next meeting so that follow-up checks can be utilized. Individual evaluation sessions can be requested at any time and annual reviews can be anticipated.

ORGANIZATION – OUR ORTHODONTIC PRACTICE

Our practice is dedicated to providing the best possible professional care and personal service to our patients. By virtue of our possession of a specialty license to practice orthodontics, our lot is to be the policy makers. Each member of the staff is essential to the success of our practice and should feel that their contributions to policy are important. Suggestions may not always be implemented but will always be given reasonable consideration. "Is there a better way?" is a question which should be uppermost in our minds.

The delegation of authority will be widely utilized in our practice. Pride in accomplishment is better manifested if personnel can be given more diverse duties and the authority to handle them in the best way they can. This stimulates team interest and promotes pride in achievement.

OFFICE WORKING HOURS

OFFICE HOURS:

Patients are normally seen in the Louisville office on a rotating weekly schedule:

Week #1: Monday, Tuesday, Wednesday
7:30 AM – 12:45 PM; 2:00 PM – 6:00 PM

Week #2: Tuesday, Wednesday, Thursday
7:30 AM – 12:45 PM; 2:00 PM – 6:00 PM

Patients are normally seen in the Bardstown office on a rotating weekly schedule:

Week #1: Monday, Tuesday
7:30 AM – 12:45 PM; 2:00 PM – 6:00 PM
Thursday
7:30 AM – 12:00 PM

Week #2 Monday, Wednesday
7:30 AM – 12:45 PM; 2:00 PM – 6:00 PM

It is extremely important that a schedule be maintained that allows full coverage at all times. The times when you are most needed are during these hours, and you are expected to keep your priorities in perspective. We will discuss any proposed changes in the schedule as far in advance as possible.

WORKING HOURS:

On regular patient days, the working hours will be:
7:00 AM – 12:45 PM; 1:45 PM – 6:00 PM

Everyone is expected to be on time. If for any reason you cannot report for work on time, please telephone the office as far in advance of your starting time as possible. Please advise the office as to when you expect to arrive, take all the time necessary to resolve your problem and make every effort to report for duty at the earliest possible time. Unsatisfactory attendance, including tardiness or leaving work early, is a particular concern in our practice and may be cause for disciplinary action.

If at any time your working hours present a temporary hardship for you, please discuss the problem with us. You are professional people and will be treated as such as long as this consideration is not abused.

PERFORMANCE REVIEW

The first performance review will be scheduled following the first three months of employment. Pertinent weaknesses and strengths will be presented in a constructive manner, and a mutual discussion of intentions and objectives will be exchanged. You are not expected to know everything about your job in three months. It is actually a time to determine if you are adequately suited to work in an orthodontic environment. Not everyone is destined to work in the health professions, and it is not in everyone's best interests to continue to pursue something in which they are not qualified or in which adequate interest is not demonstrated. Rest assured, however, that no one is hired to be fired, and every opportunity will be given for working out problems.

It is also possible that personality conflicts within the intra-office structure may dictate the need for counseling. This may be requested at any time and will be resolved immediately. This office will not tolerate petty bickering among the staff, and if a peaceful solution cannot be reached which is amicable to all parties concerned, one or both parties will be disciplined.

Annual performance reviews will be formally scheduled and usually will be held at the end of normal working hours.

SALARY

Salaries are initially based on previous experience, education, and average salaries among related health professions in the Jefferson County area. It can be presumed that you will be paid at a rate which will be at least competitive with what other offices in our community pay for your skills. Raises and bonuses are not automatic in this practice. Salary adjustments are made on the basis of performance and general attitudinal patterns. These considerations will be evaluated not less than annually, and formal sessions will be scheduled for this purpose. Economic considerations may also be a factor in determining salary levels.

Payroll deductions from your gross pay represent monies owed by you to the government for such things as taxes, social security, etc. This office has no recourse but to make these deductions. Your net take-home pay is equal to your gross salary minus all payroll deductions.

Paychecks will be issued bi-weekly on Tuesdays in Louisville, Wednesday or Thursdays in Bardstown or the last working day of every other week. Paychecks will be issued in sealed envelopes and, per a staff request, are to be kept confidential. **Any** violation of this breach of confidence will be dealt with as a violation of trust and participants are subject to dismissal.

125 FLEXIBLE SPENDING PLAN

The 125 Flexible Spending Plan is provided as a benefit to allow team members to maximize their "actual salary" by minimizing the taxes, which will be withheld from their pay. This plan, including the incurred administrative fees, is provided by Mattingly & Howell Orthodontics, P.S.C. as a courtesy to our employees and is extended unless circumstances dictate otherwise.

A team member is eligible for participation in the 125 Flexible Spending Plan after 3 months of employment. This benefit allows a team member to decide upon an amount of salary to be subtracted from each paycheck, prior to Federal, State and Social Security taxes being withheld. This money will be deposited into an account administered by Creative Retirement, Inc. and reimbursed to the team member tax free throughout the year when receipts are submitted for expenses which are included in the 125 Flexible Spending Guidelines. A comprehensive list of covered expenses will be supplied at the appropriate time and is too extensive to enumerate here, but does include child care, some insurance premiums, dental and vision costs, etc.

BENEFITS

a) Pension and Profit-Sharing Retirement Plan:
In general, a team member is eligible for the Mattingly & Howell Orthodontics, P.S.C. Retirement Plan when he/she has worked a minimum of at least 1,000 hours for one year. Currently, team members are eligible for the Mattingly & Howell Orthodontics, P.S.C. Pension Plan, which invests an amount equal to ten percent of a team member's salary in optional portfolios, which each team member directs. Also currently, a 401K matching fund plan is in existence that allows a team member to designate that up to nine percent of his/her salary be withheld and invested in certain portfolios for his/her retirement. At this time, Mattingly & Howell Orthodontics, P.S.C. is matching dollar for dollar all funding to the retirement plan up to six percent of a team member's salary. Annual summaries of retirement plan status will be made available to each team member. Currently, Creative Retirement Systems (513/741-5800) is administering the Retirement Plan and investments are handled by Fidelity Investments, Inc., Attn: Walt Schultz, 800/634-5574.

b) Life and Disability Insurance:
Mattingly & Howell Orthodontics, P.S.C. is currently contributing to the cost of a Life and Disability Insurance procurred on a group basis. For those working between 20 and 30 hours per week, $12.00 is funded per month by the corporation toward the team member's premium costs for Group Life and Disability Insurance. For those working between 30 and 40 hours per week, $15.00 is funded by the corporation per month toward the team member's premium costs for Group Life and Disability Insurance. Any premium costs over this amount funded by Mattingly & Howell Orthodontics, P.S.C. will

be deducted from the team member's weekly paycheck based on the following formula:

> Total insurance premium minus amount paid by Mattingly Orthodontics, P.S.C. = ________ x 12 months
>
> This amount divided by 26 weeks = _______ which is amount to be withheld from team member's biweekly pay.

This benefit becomes available after completion of a 90-day conditional employment period.

c) Medical and Dental Reimbursement Plan:

Medical and dental expenses incurred by each team member can be reimbursed in an amount of $75.00 per quarter. It is necessary that receipts be submitted at the end of each quarter and any additional expenses incurred over the limit may be carried over to the succeeding quarter, but may not be carried over into a new calendar year. This benefit is also available after completion of the three-month conditional employment program.

VACATIONS

Paid vacations are granted in appreciation of service to the corporation and to provide team members with a period of needed rest and relaxation. Due to the nature of an orthodontic practice, which is particularly sensitive to school schedules, it is imperative that our practice be as fully staffed as possible during these school holiday periods. Therefore, please make every effort to schedule your family vacations being sensitive to those school holidays. Also, please attempt to schedule one week of your vacation time concomitant with the week of office shut down, if at all possible.

Paid vacations after 12 months of employment are based on the number of hours worked per week. Basically, the number of hours that are worked per week will be averaged and that week's average be considered the number of hours of vacation time that a team member has earned. Two weeks paid vacation are available after 24 months of employment with the same formula applying; i.e., those averaging 36 hours per week will receive 72 hours of vacation time. However, after ten years of employment, for each additional year worked, additional vacation time equal to the average number of hours worked per day will be added to the pre-existing vacation base. This will be capped at a maximum of 120 hours, which would be obtainable for those working 40 hour weeks. Thus, if a team member averages 9 hours/day after 11 years employment, the vacation time earned would be 72 hours base plus 9 hours. After 12 years, with the same average of 9 hours per day, vacation will be 72 hours plus 18 or 90 hours. This would be capped at 15 years employment using the same prorated formula as above.

The most senior team member will have priority in the event of duplicate choices of similar vacation preference dates.

HOLIDAYS

The following holidays will be recognized as paid holidays by Mattingly & Howell Orthodontics, P.S.C.:

New Year's Day	Labor Day
Memorial Day	Thanksgiving
Fourth of July	Christmas

Other additional days or partial days may also be granted as paid holidays at the discretion of the P.S.C. Paid holidays are treated as normal working days for pay purposes.

There will be days (seminars, meetings, continuing education courses, etc.) which require that one or more of the doctors be out of the office and patients will not be scheduled. All team members are given the option of reporting for work as a normal working day or utilizing sick days or vacation time. If sick days or vacation days are exhausted, a proportionate deduction will be made from wages commensurate to the time missed.

Any changes in holiday schedules will be posted as far in advance of the proposed changes as conveniently possible.

If a holiday falls within your vacation, an additional day's salary will be provided or the choice to take an additional day's vacation at a different time will be offered. Any day other than the day immediately before or after a holiday may be chosen.

HOLIDAY PAY

Team members, excluding temporary and after school employees, will be paid their normal wage for a holiday which is celebrated on a usual work day. In the event that a holiday falls on a day which is not a typical work day, the team member will be paid for 8 hours of work. Holiday pay will be paid according to the number of hours worked during an average week. Team members who average working 30 or more hours per week will receive either 8 or 10 hours of holiday pay based on the above formula. Team members who average between 10 hours and 29 hours per week will receive 6 hours of holiday pay per holiday. Team members who average 10 hours or less per week will be paid 3 hours of holiday pay per holiday.

SICK DAYS

One work week of sick time per year is provided. For example, if a team member normally works 30 hours per week, they will be eligible for 30 hours of sick time during a year. Any absence from work after using up delegated sick time will result in proportionate loss of wages. Any unused sick time will be paid as additional salary at the end of the year. This benefit is also available after completion of the three-month conditional employment period.

PERSONAL DAYS

No time off is allotted for personal days, but time out of the office may be charged against credited sick days or vacation time. Any absence after using up delegated sick days and accrued vacation days will result in proportionate loss of wages.

LDS DAY AT THE DOWNS

The Louisville Dental Society Day at Churchill Downs is held on Friday afternoons and at the time when the office is normally not seeing patients. Those team members that wish to attend will be provided an admission ticket which includes admission, buffet luncheon and complimentary drinks. Team members are encouraged to attend in order to build rapport with other dental offices but this is not a required function.

LEAVE OF ABSENCE

A leave of absence for proper cause may be granted providing it does not seriously affect our operations and has no impact on the quality of care that we provide to our patients. Please make any requests for a leave of absence as far in advance as possible so that consideration related to maintaining your position can be explored (i.e., possible part-time or temporary coverage). Any vacation and/or sick days which you have accrued will be applied to comparable time during the leave of absence. A leave of absence will be handled in accordance with the Family Leave Act.

A leave of absence will be granted for:

a) Pregnancy Leave:
This will begin and end on the basis of the employee's personal physician's written statement regarding her ability to work. After the fifth month of pregnancy, the employee is required to periodically supply the office with a written statement from her physician regarding her ability to work and his/her estimate of the duration of her ability to work.

b) Other Reasons:
These will be considered on an individual basis and, regrettably, may not be automatic.

UNIFORM POLICY

Dress will be office logoed tops, uniform slacks (either white or the color that matches the top) and white shoes. Mattingly & Howell Orthodontics, P.S.C. will provide a $200 allowance per year to cover these items. Those employees wishing to also have matching jackets can purchase these, but would be expected to cover any costs over the $200 allowance. Receipts will need to be turned in for reimbursement on any items not purchased through the office. Mattingly & Howell Orthodontics, P.S.C. will cover the costs associated with embroidering names and logos. We request that the uniforms for all front desk personnel match each other, and all the uniforms for patient treatment personnel match each other. Treatment coordinators and lab technicians uniforms may match either front desk or floor uniforms.

MEDICAL AND DENTAL APPOINTMENTS

You are encouraged to plan personal medical and dental appointments at times which do not interfere with our normal patient treatment schedule. If your physician or dentist cannot accommodate you at those times, please attempt to make your appointments during our office lunch hour or at times which least impact our patient treatment routine.

PARKING

Parking space is available for employees' parking. It is important, though, that we all realize that the parking facility is also essential for normal patient flow. Please park only in the designated areas so that parking near the entrance is convenient for patients. Please lock your car when leaving it, as the corporation cannot be responsible for loss or theft. In the future, designated parking areas for employees may be changed depending on the types of businesses that locate in our complex. Team members are currently parking in the Dupont North lot adjacent to our main entrance to decrease congestion and maximize convenience for our patients. Parking policies may change at any time.

PERFORMANCE OF DUTIES WHEN PATIENTS ARE NOT SCHEDULED

Because of the flexibility of the profession we are in, we are able to schedule or not schedule patients at our discretion (within limits). Days when it is necessary that patients not be scheduled (meetings, seminars, continuing education courses, etc.) must be planned. When patients are not scheduled on normal working days for a team member, certain duties and responsibilities are expected to be performed. Normally, specific listing of duties and directions outlining responsibilities will not be issued. However, it is expected that your time will be wisely spent in the performance of duties benefiting the entire team. Obviously, each individual has designated responsibilities that he/she is expected to maintain (i.e. records, inventory, filing, etc.), but if these designated tasks are not sufficient to occupy your time, other tasks will be assigned. It is expected that general cleaning duties will be provided by the team members. Time when patients are not scheduled provides an excellent opportunity for general cleaning and organization. Please use this time wisely, as it is patently unfair for some employees to be consistently busy and others not to be. We are all part of a team, and the team concept stipulates that each member be willing to do his/her share plus more. When this concept is adhered to, camaraderie and friendships thrive. When it is not, the potential for resentment and animosities exists, and a breakdown in team morale can occur. Please be aware of our commitment to teamwork in this practice and make every effort to adhere to this principle.

HOUSEKEEPING

We spend more waking time in our office than at home, and there is no reason we should take less pride in our office appearance than that of our homes. It can be difficult for patients to understand how we can take pride in our work if we do not take pride in the way we look and the appearance of our work environment.

While it is not your responsibility to clean the entire facility, the participation in caring for the overall appearance of our office is expected of each team member. Drawers, cabinets, and storage areas should be neatly arranged. This also aids us in inventory control and reordering guidelines. Desk tops and work counters should be kept uncluttered and cleaned at the end of each work day. Any time that you see something that needs to be picked up, wiped off or put away, please do so without directives. Formation of an overall favorable image in the eyes of our patients, peers, and those who may potentially refer others to our office is a continuously pursued goal.

At the end of the work day, each employee is expected to make sure that everything is placed in its proper place; i.e., instruments, magazines, charts, coffee cups, etc. Sinks and mirrors should be cleaned and treatment chairs uprighted. The lounge area should be kept orderly and comfortable. This means coffee cups and lunches should not be left lying around. A clean, orderly work place instills a sense of pride, a feeling of organization and provides a favorable reflection to our patients and parents as to the quality of treatment and goals for which we strive.

PERSONAL ORTHODONTIC CARE

For those team members desiring orthodontic care, treatment will be provided free of charge as an additional benefit following 12 months of employment. This same benefit will also apply to spouses and your children. Brothers and sisters of employees will be granted a 25 percent discount. Other non-immediate members of your family such as nephews, nieces, etc., will be granted a 10 percent discount. For employees wanting Invisalign, the employee is responsible for 50 percent of the up-front cost, and Mattingly & Howell Orthodontics, PSC will pay 50 percent. If for some reason your relationship as a team member is terminated while you are in active orthodontic treatment, you and/or your family members will be requested to seek completion of your treatment with another orthodontist, and we will aid you in finding someone willing to take over the case. You and/or your family members will then be expected to make payments on a fee based on the amount of treatment remaining at the new orthodontic office.

SMOKING

The health implications of smoking shall not be taken up here. If you choose to smoke, please limit smoking to the outside of the office building, and only before and after work and during lunch hour. If you must smoke, be careful to wash your hands thoroughly and use a breath freshener before returning to work.

Smoking in the business office, reception room, lab or treatment area is not allowed.

CIVIC RESPONSIBILITIES

Any team member who is called to serve on a jury panel, or as a witness in a court proceeding, will be allowed leave of absence to serve. If you would prefer, a letter will be written in your behalf outlining your particular status in our office and requesting deferral of jury duty.

Because jury duty reimbursement may not be equal to your normal income, your jury duty payment will be supplemented to equal your normal weekly salary by the corporation for a period of two weeks. Official court documents verifying your time served and wage compensation should be submitted when you return to work.

VOTING TIME

The voting polls are usually open from early in the morning until late in the evening. It is expected that you will find time to vote either before coming to work or after you leave the office at the completion of the working day.

PERSONAL TELEPHONE CALLS

It is assumed that any personal calls you elect to make during the work day are necessary and necessarily made at that time or you would not make them. Incoming and outgoing phone calls should be brief and not cause disruption of office duties. If possible, take messages so that you can return calls at a more convenient time. Please avoid having people call you at work.

OUTSIDE EMPLOYMENT

Hopefully, the need to work a second job, after beginning employment with us, is never a consideration. Your attention, enthusiasm and energy can only be spread so far. You were employed with the consideration that your duties in this office were primary to you and any deviation in this arrangement should be discussed with team leaders.

DISCIPLINE

There may come a time when an infraction of the rules or violation of a confidence necessitates imposition of a disciplinary ruling. Team members will be given warning and, depending on the infraction, usually an opportunity to work out their problems. An attempt at fairness is paramount. If all else fails, the team member will be terminated.

If the team member feels that discipline was improperly applied, a review hearing with an independent arbitrator can be scheduled. The outcome of this hearing shall be considered final.

TERMINATION

If at any time after the three-month conditional employment program, it is necessary for your employment to be terminated, a review of your work records, time in service and other factors will be immediately performed. Obviously, if you were terminated because of a decrease in our workload, unemployment benefits may be drawn from the State Unemployment Office from an account that has been funded (at least partially) by the P.S.C. for you in this event. If, however, the nature of the infraction is such that we feel these benefits are not justifiably due you, your claim will be contested.

If you decide on your own volition that you wish to discontinue your employment with us, we request that a two-week notice be given so that adequate replacement for your position can be sought and trained.

All accrued benefits that are due you will be paid to you as quickly as possible. Funds within your Pension and Profit Sharing Plans, which have been set aside for you, normally are withdrawn, and rolled over into an IRA of your choice within 30 days.

IMMEDIATE DISMISSAL

The single largest reason for a breakdown in communication is misunderstanding. There are certain indiscretions that will not be tolerated in this office, and it is only fair that these be directly presented so as not to be misunderstood.

a) Violation of Confidential Information:

Any information that you acquire about patients and their treatment while working in this office is to remain in the office. Rumors or inappropriate stories about your fellow employees or peers are also considered a violation of a confidence. Never leave sensitive or privileged information in a position which can be observed by a casual visitor or patient. Some work-related stories and incidents would be better left unrelated to friends and spouses. Please use discretion when talking about the office or your fellow workers. Your salary and personal benefits are also confidential and discussion about your salary with other employees is considered to be a violation of confidential information.

b) Embezzlement of Funds, Equipment or Supplies:

Mistakes can be made by anyone, but any proven deliberate mishandling of corporate monies or supplies will result in immediate dismissal and in filing of criminal charges.

c) Fraudulent Forgery of Documents:

If any deliberate forgery for improper reasons can be proven, immediate dismissal will result.

d) Improper Use of Controlled Drugs or Alcohol:

The improper use of controlled drugs or alcohol while on duty can also result in immediate dismissal.

e) Conviction of a Felonious Charge:

If you are convicted of a felony, your work here will be terminated. Remember that your behavior reflects on your work and reputation. A serious error in judgment can live with you forever.

TEMPORARY EMPLOYMENT PERSONNEL

Certain circumstances require employment status to be considered temporary (Students from Jefferson State Vocational Program, High School Coop. Students, etc.). These same circumstances determine work hours, whether salaries are paid and length of employment depending upon your specific situation. If salaries are paid, this salary is to be considered the entire compensation from the corporation and it should be understood that other benefits enjoyed by permanent team members are not necessarily applicable for temporary employees. This includes Pension Funds, 125 Cafeteria Plan, 401K Matching Retirement Plan, Life and Disability Insurance, Uniform Allowance, and Vacation and Sick Days Compensation.

All other aspects of this Office Policy Manual are pertinent to Temporary Employment Personnel. This includes adherence to regular work hours, as dictated by your particular situation, personal appearance guidelines, policies regarding housekeeping, smoking, personal phone calls, parking, and sexual harassment. A special note should be made concerning the importance of confidentiality. This is a professional office and any information that you may acquire regarding patients, other employees, or doctors during your employment with this Corporation should be held in the strictest of confidence. This Manual spells out certain situations, which would result in immediate termination of employment and possibly prosecution. Please pay particular attention to the importance of these matters.

We want you to know that every member of our team will do everything possible to make your temporary employment as enjoyable as possible. Please advise us of any questions or problems that may arise during your employment with Mattingly & Howell Orthodontics, P.S.C.

Appendix B

Mattingly & Howell Orthodontics, P.S.C.
Office Policy Against Sexual Harassment

General:

As an equal opportunity employer, the offices of Mattingly & Howell Orthodontics, P.S.C. are committed to providing our employees with a workplace that is free of sexual harassment. Acts of sexual harassment will not be tolerated.

To help enforce this policy, it will be prominently posted and reviewed with every employee as part of the indoctrination.

Violators of this policy may be subject to discipline, up to and including termination. Employees will not be subjected to retaliation for complaining of harassment.

Definition of Sexual Harassment:

Sexual harassment is a form of discrimination prohibited by Title VII of the Civil Rights Act. It can occur in any of several forms, including unwelcome sexual advances, and other verbal or physical conduct of a sexual nature when:

1. Submission to such conduct is made either explicitly a term or condition of an individual's employment.
2. Submission to, or rejection of, such conduct by a person is used as the basis of, or factor in, an employment decision affecting the person.
3. Such conduct has the purpose, or effect of, unreasonably interfering with a person's work performance or creating an intimidating, hostile, or offensive working environment.

Personal behavior or language that is acceptable to one person may be offensive to another. Everyone must use sound personal judgment as to how their actions may affect others.

Examples of Sexual Harassment

1. Off-color jokes.
2. Repeated unsolicited sexual flirtations.
3. Advances or propositions.
4. Continued or repeated verbal comments or physical actions of a sexual nature.
5. Graphic comments about a person's body.
6. Sexually degrading words to describe a person.
7. Touching, patting, or pinching.
8. Display in the workplace of sexually suggestive objects or pictures.

What is Not Sexual Harassment

1. Isolated comments of a sexual nature.
2. Conduct between consenting persons.
3. Actions arising out of current personal or social relationships where no coercion is involved.
4. Occasional compliments of a non-sexual nature.

Summary:

No employee need submit to any unwelcome advances of a sexual nature.

Under no circumstances will rejection of such advances adversely affect the length or condition of your employment here.

Complaints:

All complaints of sexual harassment will be investigated.

Any employee who thinks he or she has been the victim of sexual harassment should report promptly the alleged discrimination to Dr. John Mattingly, Dr. Chris Mattingly, or Dr. Chris Howell.

Dr. John Mattingly, Dr. Chris Mattingly, or Dr. Chris Howell are responsible for thoroughly investigating the matter.

Dr. John Mattingly, Dr. Chris Mattingly, or Dr. Chris Howell will discuss the matter with both parties and question all employees who know about the incident in question or similar situations. The complaint, investigative steps, findings, and disposition should be thoroughly documented.

After the investigation is completed, Dr. John Mattingly, Dr. Chris Mattingly, or Dr. Chris Howell will take appropriate corrective action.

Although the office normally expects to resolve complaints internally, employees should be aware that they are entitled to file complaints of sexual harassment with the Equal Opportunity Employment Commission or other appropriate government agency.

Harassment by Non-Employees:

If an employee feels that he or she has been harassed by a vendor, maintenance person, or other non-employee, the employee should bring the matter to the attention of Dr. John Mattingly, Dr. Chris Mattingly, or Dr. Chris Howell.

Appendix C

PATIENT SATISFACTION SURVEY

MATTINGLY ORTHODONTICS, PSC

Dr. John B. Mattingly, D.M.D., M.S.
Dr. Chris Mattingly, D.M.D., M.S.
Dr. Chris Howell, D.M.D., M.S.
Louisville and Bardstown, Kentucky

1. What is your relationship to this office?
   Patient_____ Family member of patient_____

2. What is your age group?
   5-10 years_____ 11-14_____ 15-18_____ 18-21_____ over 21_____

3. What is the length of time you have been coming to this office?
   <1 year_____ <18 months_____ <2 years_____ <3 years_____ >3 years_____

	ANALYSIS RATING	EXCELLENT	GOOD	FAIR	POOR
4.	Procedure/policy for scheduling appointments?	1	2	3	4
5.	Telephone courtesy and procedures?	1	2	3	4
6.	Comfort of reception area?	1	2	3	4
7.	Waiting time after arrival?	1	2	3	4
8.	Overall office appearance, organization, and cleanliness?	1	2	3	4
9.	Appearance of Staff?	1	2	3	4
10.	Friendliness/helpfulness of receptionist and front office staff?	1	2	3	4
11.	Friendliness/helpfulness of treatment assistants and doctors?	1	2	3	4
12.	Quality of orthodontic care provided by this office?	1	2	3	4
13.	Sterilization procedures?	1	2	3	4
14.	Explanation of progress and procedures during treatment?	1	2	3	4
15.	Explanation/help with financial arrangements?	1	2	3	4

16. How long do you typically wait to be seen after you arrive for an appointment?
    0-5 minutes_____ 5-15 minutes_____ 16-30 minutes_____ 31-45 minutes _____
    >45 minutes_____

17. Would you recommend our office to others? Yes_____ No_____
    Don't Know_____

18. What is the one thing you like best about our office?

19. What is the one thing you would change about our office?

20. Do you have any additional comments to clarify your responses to this questionnaire?

Survey adapted and modified from *Ormco Corp. prototype.
(Ormco Corp., 1332 South Lone Hill Ave., Glendora, Cal. 91740)

Appendix D

Statement printed in VIEWPOINT

Sub-heading LETTERS
ADA News April 5, 2004

February 5, 2004

We as members of the American Dental Association are a family of believers, united in one spirit, and dedicated to the treatment and care of our patients. Ours may be the only profession in creation that works daily toward making itself extinct. Preventive dentistry is more than a catchy phrase – it is a philosophy that we all subscribe to. The general public is well aware that dentistry's position on brushing, sugar intake, flossing, smokeless tobacco, etc. is exclusively for the benefit of the public and is not self-serving.

Let us never forget that what most people consider dentistry's greatest contribution to our patients – fluoridation of public water supplies – was not accomplished by buying access to legislators so we could convince them of the merits of the program. Rather, the conviction that the public good was being served and the power of a unified front is what influenced legislators in local communities and sent a message to all legislators that dentistry's commitment to our patients and the common good was paramount. Nor was this selfless campaign lost on the general public who for years have rated dentistry at or near the top of the most trusted professions in Gallup Polls. Somewhere along the line, however, it appears that dentistry has lost its sense of mission and now the cries of less government, less regulations, less taxes but more programs and more public dollars for dental needs appear, at least, paradoxical to the public we serve. Not surprisingly, our trust ratings are slipping and dentistry is perceived as having elected to follow other professions along the path of "what can you do for me?"

Dentistry needs to re-evaluate our mission. The first step in this re-evaluation should be to discontinue attempting to influence legislation by buying legislators. Our legacy of selfless actions over the years has brought our profession to where it is. It was not built on supporting the "underlying cause of the public's disgust with politics" (U. S. Senator John McCain on announcing his candidacy for President, Jan. 30, 1999).

At a time when the very moral fiber of our government is threatened by the influence of special interest money pursuing access to legislation favorable to its cause, it appears that the American Dental Association has lost sight of the mission of our organization. In an attempt to gain access to legislators so that dentistry's messages can be favorably received, it has become standard policy to employ lobbyists to ply legislators with monies to influence their vote. This practice has become widespread by associations, corporations, unions and special interest groups of all denominations resulting in conflicting bidding wars of benefit primarily to the lobbyists, legislators, and largest contributors.

The very practice of seeking to buy influence at best hints of impropriety and could possibly lead to corruption. It is difficult for me to buy into the logic that it's the right thing to do because everyone else is doing it. Each of us as individuals, and collectively as our Association, must take responsibility for our actions and their results. The bottom line is that we are attempting to curry favor with legislators by contributing money in hopes of securing legislation favorable to our special interests. It is wrong, we know it is wrong, and yet we have been caught up in this "what can you do for me" rat race.

No government can continue to operate under such a system. It completely disenfranchises those without funds. The First Amendment guarantees free speech and as long as those with the most money have the loudest voice, this constitutional right is being denied.

If the younger generation that is presently so disgusted with the current process that they stay away from the polls in droves is ever to develop a trust in our political system, significant changes must be made in the process.

There are alternatives to PACs and soft money. Public financing of campaigns is being utilized in several states and others are exploring it. Public financing forces candidates to discuss the issues and eliminate the continuous need for focusing on fund raising for election or re-election.

The ADA grass roots movement has the potential to be one of the most successful and beneficial programs in existence. It can be particularly effective as long as the participants are convinced that the merits of their efforts are for the proper purpose, and the stigma of attempting to influence legislation with money is removed.

If you share my concerns about current ADA policy of contributing money to legislators, let your Trustee know so that at least the appropriateness of such a policy can be reconsidered. ADA Trustees are hard-working, well-meaning representatives of their constituents and need to be made aware of members' concerns about this issue.

Sincerely,

John B. Mattingly, D.M.D.

July 1, 2003

Board of Trustees
American Association of Orthodontists
401 N. Lindbergh Boulevard
St. Louis, Missouri 63141-7816

Gentlemen,

I have recently received my statement for membership dues dated for the time period of 8/01/03 through 5/31/04 and, as I have done so systematically for the past 32 years, I am forwarding a check for AAO, Constituent (SAO) and Component (KAO) dues. I have never questioned the amount of the dues nor any assessment that was mandated by the AAO House of Delegates. I did so because I believed that we as members of the American Association of Orthodontists (and the American Dental Association as well) are a family united in one spirit and dedicated to the treatment and care of our patients. I have believed the profession of orthodontics was never about us, but about the people we served and almost all energies were devoted to collaborative sharing of knowledge and experiences allowing our profession to develop into the most accessible, affordable, appreciated profession in existence We have been truly blessed.

I am now entering the twilight of my orthodontic career. I see some storm clouds on the horizon … a number of which I can do nothing about. But one of the major concerns I have is the practice of buying "access" to legislators so we can convince them of the merits of a program we support. This practice has become widespread by associations, corporations, unions and special interest groups of all denominations, resulting in conflicting bidding wars of benefit primarily to lobbyists, legislators and the largest contributors. Our leaders have championed the cause of getting the government out of our offices while petitioning government for a larger share of government entitlement programs. This disparity fools only fools. How can someone who didn't wear rubber gloves and used Zephryn Chloride Cold sterilization until OSHA mandated differently, ever believe that all government regulations are against us personally? Anytime that money is used to buy legislative influence for a special interest benefit, it corroded the doctor-patient relationships which we have worked so long to develop.

I have taken the liberty of enclosing a letter that I sent to the American Dental Association Publishing Company, the publisher of "The Journal of the American Dental Association" further explaining my concerns and requesting that it be printed either as an editorial or as a letter to the editor. The letter was never printed.*

As you will notice, the check for my tripartite dues does not include the $16.74 (fee to lobbyists and contributions to legislators) that the AAO has estimated will be "allocated to programs and activities necessary for the preservation and promotion of the interests of patients and the specialty". The $16.74, obviously, I can afford and I surely would never challenge whatever amount of funds for promoting the interest of our patients or specialty. However, I do challenge the practice of buying legislators and therefore in good conscience cannot participate in something that I feel contributes to the moral erosion of our society.

This influence of money on government cannot go on forever. It will change ... and I would hope to see the American Association of Orthodontists assume a leadership role in publicly announcing that they find the practice objectionable and refuse to be a party to this "legalized corruption" ... Or, the low road is the most heavily traveled and the most popular ... for the moment!

Sincerely,

John B. Mattingly, D.M.D.

---

* The letter was subsequently printed - ADA News April 5, 2004

Letter that I had planned to send out to all orthodontists in U.S. and Canada but was denied access to mailing labels that the American Association of Orthodontists sells to vendors.

December, 2003

Re: What Price Dissension?

Dear Doctor,

Did you ever wonder about the consequences when you stand up for what you believe is right? Do you consider the ramifications of a dissenting voice in the face of an intimidating majority? Each of us in the profession of orthodontics has made tough choices, some on a daily basis. Each of us has experienced the concerns of the threat to the viability of our profession as we have responded to capitation programs, managed service buyouts, and the overlap in scope of practice intrusions. We have done so by uniting in a cohesive body focused in overcoming adversity because we knew that we were doing the right things. Historically, the professions of dentistry and orthodontics have demonstrated selfless dedication to the service of our patients and the betterment of our communities. It was no accident that the profession of dentistry had consistently ranked in the top three most trusted professions in Gallup Polls conducted in our country.

My brothers and sisters in the dental family and orthodontic profession, it appears that somewhere along the line, we are losing our sense of mission. The cries of less government, less regulations, less taxes but pleas for more programs and more dollars for dental needs are appearing, at least, paradoxical to the public we serve. Not surprisingly, our trust ratings are slipping and our profession is perceived as having elected to follow other professions along the path of "What's in it for me?"

In June, 2003, I received an invoice for AAO dues which also included Constituent (SAO) and Component (KAO) dues. As I have systematically done for 32 years, I forwarded a check within the next week to AAO. Only this time, I sent a letter (copy enclosed) which notified the AAO Board that I did not support AAO-PAC's attempt to influence legislators with money and withheld $16.74 (fee to lobbyists and contributions to legislators). I was summarily contacted by my Constituent Trustee asking me to reconsider and notifying me that the AAO Board would be forced to make a ruling on my status if I failed to comply. A copy of the Board notification is also enclosed.

I subsequently called the AAO Bulletin and requested that I be given an opportunity to present my position on the matter of the influence of special interest money pursuing legislation favorable to its specific interests. I suggested that a point-counterpoint forum be presented and representatives from AAO-PAC present their position. I had been advised that the AAO Bulletin was an autonomous publication and was not under the directorship of the AAO Board but was advised by the Editor of the Bulletin that Board Approval would be necessary and that my proposal would be an AAO Board Agenda item at the November Board meeting. When I called to check on the decision of the Board, I was notified that the AAO Board had not yet met but the proposal would not be going to the Board as the AAO President had made a Presidential Decision that no forum would be provided.

Hence, my position is this: After 32 years of membership in the American Association of Orthodontists, having served as President of the Southern Association of Orthodontists, an eight-year term on the AAO Council on Membership, Ethics and Judicial Concerns (3 years as Chairman) a two term presidency of the Kentucky Orthodontic Association, a term as President of the Louisville Dental Society and a term as President of the Kentucky Dental Association, along with many other councils and committees during this time, I find myself with my membership revoked in an organization that I have both supported and cherished over the years because I have refused to pay $16.74 (fee to lobbyists and contributions to legislators). My request to voice my concerns has been denied and I find no recourse other than to share my story by individual letter to my colleagues and peers in the only manner I see remaining.

When the speaker at our constituent meeting where we honor our most deserving recipients, the leaders of our profession, clinicians, researchers, educators (the Jarabak Award, the Distinguished Service Award, etc.) is a Washington Lobbyist and the scheduled featured speaker at the 2004 AAO Annual Session Breakfast is Bill O'Reilly, I submit to you, my brothers and sisters, that the direction that our profession is taking is a tenuous one. It is never easy to stand with a position that runs counter to the flow, but I sincerely believe that it is the "right thing to do", and I can do no less.

So, why do I send out a letter of this type to orthodontists all over the country? Am I truly a Don Quixote, well-intentioned but fighting windmills? Or, is there a concern out there in the hinterland that we are losing our sense of mission and we need to refocus on what brought us to where we are. We truly belong to the greatest profession known to mankind, respected by our peers, and loved by our patients... It is ours to lose!!

I would like to see the AAO and ADA return to the High Road – make a public announcement that our organizations consider attempting to purchase legislation favorable to our interests reprehensible and dare any legislator to deny us access if the potential care of our patients is ever compromised. It is not only the right thing to do, it is the only thing to do.

What can you do? If you share my concerns about the direction our professional organizations are taking, call or email your trustee demanding that your dues be used only for purposes other than influencing legislators with money. Such a message does not mean that a Governmental Affairs Committee cannot exist, but the directive that no monies are to be offered will alert legislators that we are taking the High Road, proud of our relationships with our patients and our concern for their behalf, and refuse to buy access when advocating for their interests. Again it is the right thing to do!

> **"Focus on enriching, rather than getting rich, on serving rather than being served; what you do for yourselves dies with you, what you do for others is immortal!"**
>
> ***Anonymous***

• •

The writer can be reached by email to jandjmatt@insightbb.com
and would appreciate your comments, pro or con.

BUY A SHARE OF THE FUTURE IN YOUR COMMUNITY

These certificates make great holiday, graduation and birthday gifts that can be personalized with the recipient's name. The cost of one S.H.A.R.E. or one square foot is $54.17. The personalized certificate is suitable for framing and will state the number of shares purchased and the amount of each share, as well as the recipient's name. The home that you participate in "building" will last for many years and will continue to grow in value.

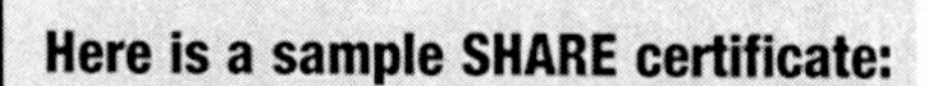

Here is a sample SHARE certificate:

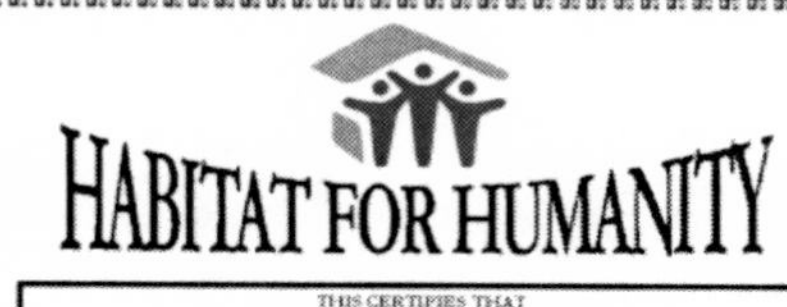

THIS CERTIFIES THAT

YOUR NAME HERE

HAS INVESTED IN A HOME FOR A DESERVING FAMILY

1985-2005

TWENTY YEARS OF BUILDING FUTURES IN OUR COMMUNITY ONE HOME AT A TIME

1200 SQUARE FOOT HOUSE @ $65,000 = $54.17 PER SQUARE FOOT

This certificate represents a tax deductible donation. It has no cash value.

YES, I WOULD LIKE TO HELP!

I support the work that Habitat for Humanity does and I want to be part of the excitement! As a donor, I will receive periodic updates on your construction activities but, more importantly, I know my gift will help a family in our community realize the dream of homeownership. ***I would like to SHARE in your efforts against substandard housing in my community!*** *(Please print below)*

PLEASE SEND ME ___________ SHARES at $54.17 EACH = $ $___________

In Honor Of: ____

Occasion: *(Circle One)* *HOLIDAY* *BIRTHDAY* *ANNIVERSARY*

OTHER: ____

Address of Recipient: ____

Gift From: _______________ ***Donor Address:*** ________________________________

Donor Email: ____

I AM ENCLOSING A CHECK FOR $ $_____________ PAYABLE TO HABITAT FOR HUMANITY <u>OR</u> PLEASE CHARGE MY VISA OR MASTERCARD *(CIRCLE ONE)*

Card Number ________________________________ Expiration Date: ____________

Name as it appears on Credit Card __________________ Charge Amount $ ____________

Signature ____

Billing Address ____

Telephone # Day __________________________ Eve __________________________

PLEASE NOTE: Your contribution is tax-deductible to the fullest extent allowed by law.

Habitat for Humanity • P.O. Box 1443 • Newport News, VA 23601 • 757-596-5553

www.HelpHabitatforHumanity.org

Breinigsville, PA USA
18 August 2009
222451BV00003B/4/P

9 781600 375569